Workbook

The Administrative
Dental Assistant

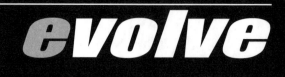

To access your student Resources, visit:

http://evolve.elsevier.com/Gaylor/ada/

Evolve ® Student Learning Resources for *Gaylor: The Administrative Dental Assistant, Second Edition,* reaches beyond the textbook with these additional features:

Student Resources

- **Crossword Puzzles**
  Review key terms and concepts through these interactive exercices.

- **Weblinks**
  Instant access to hundreds of related online resources.

- **Continually Updated CDT Code**
  Dental terminology index revised whenever new codes are released.

http://evolve.elsevier.com/Gaylor/ada

Workbook

The Administrative Dental Assistant

2nd edition

Linda J. Gaylor, RDA
Education Programs Consultant
California Department of Education
Sacramento, California

SAUNDERS

ELSEVIER

SAUNDERS
ELSEVIER

11830 Westline Industrial Drive
St. Louis, Missouri 63146

WORKBOOK FOR THE ADMINISTRATIVE DENTAL
ASSISTANT, SECOND EDITION

ISBN 13: 978-1-4160-2565-8
ISBN 10: 1-4160-2565-0

Copyright © 2007, 2000 by Saunders, an imprint of Elsevier Inc.

All rights reserved. No part of this publication may be reproduced or transmitted in any form or by any
means, electronic or mechanical, including photocopying, recording, or any information storage and retrieval
system, without permission in writing from the publisher. Although for mechanical reasons all pages of this
publication are perforated, only those pages imprinted with an Elsevier Inc. copyright notice are intended for
removal.

Permissions may be sought directly from Elsevier's Health Sciences Rights Department in Philadelphia, PA,
USA: phone: (+1) 215 239 3804, fax: (+1) 215 239 3805, e-mail: healthpermissions@elsevier.com. You may
also complete your request on-line via the Elsevier homepage (http://www.elsevier.com), by selecting
'Customer Support' and then 'Obtaining Permissions'.

Notice

Neither the Publisher nor the Author assumes any responsibility for any loss or injury and/or damage to
persons or property arising out of or related to any use of the material contained in this book. It is the responsibility of the treating practitioner, relying on independent expertise and knowledge of the patient, to
determine the best treatment and method of application for the patient.

The Publisher

ISBN-13: 978-1-4160-2565-8
ISBN-10: 1-4160-2565-0

Publishing Director: Linda Duncan
Senior Editor: John Dolan
Developmental Editor: John Dedeke
Editorial Assistant: Marcia Bunda
Publishing Services Manager: Pat Joiner
Senior Project Manager: Karen M. Rehwinkel
Design Direction: Julia Dummitt
Cover Designer: Julia Dummitt

Printed in the United States of America
Last digit is the print number: 9 8 7 6 5 4

Working together to grow
libraries in developing countries

www.elsevier.com | www.bookaid.org | www.sabre.org

ELSEVIER   BOOK AID International   Sabre Foundation

Introduction

The Workbook, CD-ROM, and Dentrix Software Demo have been designed to help you perfect the skills and objectives outlined in *The Administrative Dental Assistant*. To help you achieve these objectives, the workbook includes the following:

- **Chapter Introductions** that briefly state the key concept and goals of each chapter.
- **Objectives** that identify the concepts and skills that are necessary to master the goal of each chapter.
- **Exercises** that ask questions that will require you to list information, identify key concepts, and match terms with their definitions. Short-answer questions will direct you to solve problems and sequence activities. It is the intention of the exercises to help you achieve the objectives in the textbook by providing a means to study, work with others, and develop necessary skills.
- **Activity Exercises** will help you apply information learned in order to complete tasks that will be similar to tasks you will encounter as an administrative dental assistant. The activities will require you to use information assembled in one activity to complete the next task. It is very important that you complete the tasks in the order in which they are presented. Before moving on to the next task, you should verify the correctness of the completed task. It will be helpful if you refer to information identified in the "Anatomy of..." figures and procedures outlined in the textbook. **Remember:** The tasks are sequenced and must be completed in the order presented.
- **Dentrix Exercises** will introduce you to a ***real world*** dental practice management software. Dentrix is a leader in dental practice management software and dental office technology integration. The CD provided in this workbook is a fully executable version of Dentrix 11. During **tutorial practice** you will be directed through a series of exercises that demonstrates the basic functions of the software. In addition, you will be guided through specific tasks and given the opportunity to enter data. During **independent practice** you will have the chance to enter patient data, create patient files, develop treatment plans, generate insurance claim forms, and perform basic daily procedures used in most dental practices. The tutorial and independent practice follow some of the same exercises identified in the Activity Exercises and are designed to be used concurrently. As an added resource, the software includes an extensive *Help* menu and the ***Dentrix 11 Users Guide.***
- **The Administrative Dental Assistant CD-ROM** is bound in the back of the textbook. The interactive CD-ROM has been designed to simulate a day in the life of an administrative dental assistant, and you can begin exploring elements of the CD from the beginning. In the program, each day of the week increases in difficulty and introduces new concepts. Concepts are directly related to material in the textbook (you may find the exercises to have more significance after completing chapters 3 through 15).

I hope that you will find the textbook and the accompanying material useful in pursuing an exciting career as a member of a dental healthcare team.

Linda J. Gaylor

Contents

Introduction to Dentrix Practice Management Software

Included with each copy of *Workbook for The Administrative Dental Assistant Student* is a complimentary copy of Dentrix practice management software.

This program allows you to explore all of the basic features of Dentrix, and to perform the software exercises listed through the workbook.* The software must be installed on your computer to work. This introduction provides instructions for installing the software on individual and network PCs, as well as a brief overview of the five Dentrix modules.

DENTRIX USER'S MANUAL

It is recommended that users download and review the *Dentrix 11 User's Guide* from the *Dentrix 11* CD-ROM. To do this, insert the CD-ROM in your computer and select My Computer from the desktop. Open the CD-ROM drive and select the Documentation folder. From this folder, open the Dentrix 11 User's Guide.

NOTE: *It* **will not** *be necessary to print the full Dentrix 11 User's Guide,* although during Dentrix exercises you may want to print selected sections of the guide. *Please note that the document is very large and totals almost 1150 pages.*

WARNING: Check your computer application for the correct procedure to print a range of pages or ask your instructor for directions

INSTALLATION

System Requirements

Dentrix requires:

- Windows 2000 or Windows XP Professional; the latest service pack must be installed for all operating systems
- A minimum of 20 GB of free hard disk space (for Document Center storage) on the server (or single-user system); a minimum of 1 GB free on each workstation

For best results, Dentrix recommends:

- Genuine Intel Pentium IV or faster computer
- 256 MB of RAM (512 MB on servers)
- 17″ or larger monitors (set to 1024 × 68 resolution with 32-bit color)

Notes:

- Microsoft Windows® must be installed before you install Dentrix.
- Windows® NT 4.0 and Windows® 98 SE have been tested but may not be compatible with some functions within Dentrix 11.0. For specific functions that may not be compatible, please see the Dentrix System Requirements.
- System requirements are subject to change according to current computer industry standards. For complete system recommendations and requirements, please contact Dentrix and request current "System Requirements" and "Networking Guide" documents by calling 1-800-DENTRIX (336-8749) or visiting www.dentrix.com.

Before Installing

The information contained in this section can be vital to a smooth installation of Dentrix 11. Read this section carefully before beginning the installation. If you are installing Dentrix on a networked system, you will need to complete the installation process on each workstation. You should install Dentrix on the file server first (the system where the data files will be stored).

---

* The version of Dentrix included with this workbook is a multi-user lockdown version. It includes access to all of the core Dentrix features but does not enable the user to change or customize practice information. To obtain practice customization capability, please purchase the commercial version of Dentrix by visiting www.dentrix.com.

Introduction to Dentrix Practice Management Software

Dedicated Servers

If your network has a dedicated file server (a system used only to store data and is not used for data entry), do not install Dentrix on the dedicated server. Instead, install Dentrix on the first workstation as if it is the file server. Be sure to point the paths for the Data Files and Letter Templates to the dedicated server's hard drive.

Installing Dentrix 11

If you are installing on a networked system, the following steps should be completed on the file server first.

1. Insert CD-ROM

Insert the Dentrix 11 CD-ROM into your CD-ROM drive. If your CD-ROM drive is equipped with AutoStart technology, the Install Startup screen will appear within a few seconds. Click the Dentrix 11 option and proceed to step 4.

If the Install Startup screen does not appear, you should complete steps 2 and 3.

2. Click Start | Run (Optional)

Click on the Windows® Start button and then choose Run. The Run dialog box will appear.

3. Type D:\Disk1\Setup in the Command Line (Optional)

Type D:\Disk\Setup in the command line (if your CD-ROM drive is identified by a letter other than D, substitute that letter for D). Click the OK button to begin the installation. The Installation Screen will appear for several seconds, followed by a Welcome screen.

Introduction to Dentrix Practice Management Software

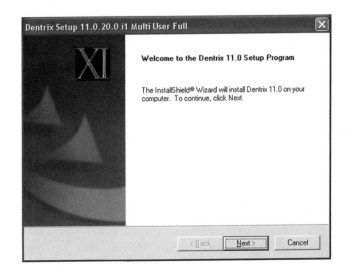

4. Click Next

Read the information contained on the Welcome screen and click the Next button to continue. If you are upgrading from a previous version of Dentrix, a message will appear stating that a backup is strongly recommended before continuing. If you have a valid backup of your data, click Yes to continue. (If not, click No and the installation will end. You may begin the installation again after a backup is completed.)

5. Click Yes

The Software License Agreement screen will appear. Read the Software License Agreement. If you agree with the terms contained in the agreement, click the Yes button. The installation will continue. (If you do not agree with the terms, click No and the installation will be terminated).

6. Select Station Type

If you are installing on the local file server or across the network to a dedicated file server (the computer that will store the data files), highlight Server Install. If you are installing on a workstation, highlight Workstation Install. Click Next to continue.

Introduction to Dentrix Practice Management Software

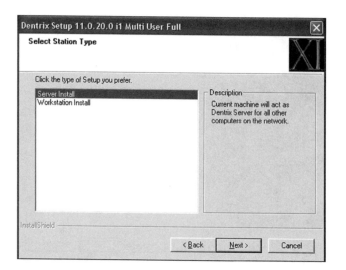

7. Check System Requirements

A message will appear asking if you want to check your computer against Dentrix System Requirements. It is recommended that you click Yes to make sure your system can handle the Dentrix practice management system.

8. Enter Serial Number

Enter your name, the name of the company, and your serial number (023822 – DEC80V89). Click Next to continue (you must enter a valid serial number to continue).

9. Select Destination Folder

Make certain the destination folder is correct. By default, Dentrix will select C:\Program Files\Dentrix for new users and the existing program directory for upgrading users. Click the Next button to continue. The Edit Default Directories dialog box appears.

Dentrix Setup 11.0.20.0 i1 Multi User Full

Select Destination

Setup will install Dentrix 11.0 in the following folder.

To install to this folder, click Next. To install to a different folder, click Browse and select another folder.

Destination Folder

C:\Program Files\Dentrix\   [Browse...]

InstallShield

[< Back] [Next >] [Cancel]

NOTE: *If you are upgrading from a previous version, a message will inform you that the rebuild utility must be run. Click OK to run the rebuild. Click OK upon completion of the rebuild utility. A rebuild must be successful before the installation can continue. Contact Dentrix Support if errors are encountered when running a Rebuild.*

10. **Edit Default Directories**

The Edit Default Directories dialog box allows you to make certain that Dentrix installs to the appropriate directories. By default, the recommended directories will be selected for new users. Current Settings will be selected for upgrading users.

Explanations of the different directories are listed below:

Dentrix Setup 11.0.20.0 i1 Multi User Full

Edit Default Directories

Please select the locations for the following Dentrix components:

Data Files Folder

C:\Program Files\Dentrix\Data   [Browse...]

Template Files Folder

C:\Program Files\Dentrix\Doc   [Browse...]

Tutor Files Folder

C:\Program Files\Dentrix\Tutor   [Browse...]

InstallShield

[< Back] [Next >] [Cancel]

- **Data Files Folder:** Patient information files. For networked versions, these files should only be installed on the file server.
- **Template Files Folder:** Letter templates Dentrix uses to create letters. Templates should only be installed on the file server.
- **Tutor Files Folder:** Information files used to practice while learning Dentrix. Tutor files should be installed on each workstation.

When you are certain the destination directories are correct, click the Next button. The Select Features dialog box will appear.

11. Select Components to Install

The Select Program Folder dialog box allows you to choose which files you want to install. The list of subcomponents changes according to which component is highlighted.

NOTE: *If you are installing on a workstation, certain components and subcomponents will not be available for selection.*

- **Program Files:** This option will install the program files and must be selected if you wish to install Dentrix or a Dentrix upgrade.

- **Data Files:** *New users should select this option.* **Upgrading users should NOT select this option.** By choosing this option, any existing patient information will be overwritten and lost.

  WARNING: *Do NOT check this option if you have previously entered information in Dentrix.*

- **Tutor Files:** You can choose to install helpful tutorial files to assist in learning Dentrix basics. See the Tutorial section of the Dentrix 11 User's Guide for more information. It is recommended that networked users install the tutorial files on each workstation. Upgrading users, who have installed the tutorial files previously, should replace the tutorial files when installing an update. *Please note: Tutorials will be assigned during the Dentrix Exercises section of the workbook.*

- **Letter Files:** *New users should select this option.* **Upgrading users should NOT select this option.** Selecting this option will cause your existing Dentrix letters to be overwritten. Any customizing of letters you may have performed will be lost.

- **Setup Files:** This will install the setup files necessary to install Dentrix at a later time if needed. If you are installing on the files server, this option should be checked if you are a new user or an upgrading user.

Once all of the correct components and subcomponents are selected, click the Next button to continue the installation.

12. Select Program Folder

"Dentrix" will automatically be selected for the Program Folder. This will be the name of the folder where the Dentrix modules will be located. If you wish to change this folder, type the desired name or select one from a list. Click the Next button to continue.

NOTE: *If you are upgrading from a previous version, the conversion utility will launch here. Once the conversion is completed, click Continue to advance the installation.*

13. Complete Installation

When the installation program has finished loading the Dentrix software, the Setup Complete window will appear, informing you that the installation is complete. Click the Finish button to complete the installation.

Installing Dentrix Over a Network

Once Dentrix 11 has been installed on the File Server you can quickly install Dentrix 11 on the workstations by accessing the Setup files from the server. This installation method allows you to install multiple stations without using the CD-ROM.

Before following any of the instructions below, be sure that your network has been properly installed and configured by a System Technician. Refer to the Dentrix Networking Guide (available by calling 1-800-DENTRIX) for recommendations.

NOTE: *Before completing the instructions below, there should be a drive mapped to the File Server. Dentrix recommends that the same drive letter be used for each workstation (i.e., "M").*

1. Choose Start | Run

Click the Windows® Start button located on your desktop and choose Run.

2. Type M:\Program Files\Dentrix\Setup\Setup.exe

Type M:\Program Files\Dentrix\Setup\Setup.exe on the command line. ('M' represents the drive letter used to map the File Server.) The Installation Setup screen appears for several seconds followed by the Welcome screen.

3. Click Next

Click the Next button. The Software License Agreement dialog box will appear.

4. Click Yes

Click the Yes button to agree to the Software License Agreement. The Select Station Type dialog box will appear.

5. Select Station Type

Highlight Workstation Install and click Next.

6. Check System Requirements

A message will appear asking if you want to check your computer against Dentrix System Requirements. It is recommended that you click Yes to make sure this workstation can handle the Dentrix practice management systems.

7. Destination Directory

The destination directory is the location where the Dentrix program will be installed. Be sure this is the correct location and hit Next.

8. **Edit Default Directories**

   The Edit Default Directories dialog box will appear. The Data and Template paths should be pointed to the network drive. Once you are certain the default directories are correct, click Next.

9. **Select Components**

   The Select Components to Install dialog box will appear. Choose Program Files, Tutor Files, and Setup Files. Click the Next button.

10. **Select Program Folder**

    Enter the name of the Program Folder or select one from the list. Dentrix will automatically enter or select "Dentrix" for the Program Folder. This will be the name of the folder where the Dentrix modules will be located. Click the Next button to continue.

11. **Complete Installation**

    When the installation program has finished loading the Dentrix software, the Setup Complete screen will appear. Click Finish to complete the installation. Repeat for any other workstations on the network.

DENTRIX OVERVIEW

As a clinical and practice management software system, Dentrix manages a variety of information, including patient demographics, clinical details, and production analysis. To simplify the process of entering and finding data, the Dentrix program is divided into five separate modules that each manage specific types of information.

Family File

The Family File module manages patients' demographic and insurance information. From this module you will keep track of a patient's name, address, employer, insurance information, notes, continuing care, and other important information.

Patient Chart

The Patient Chart module manages the clinical information for patients. Using common textbook symbols, the Chart lets you post existing, completed, and recommended procedures. Additionally, the Chart helps you to keep extensive and detailed notes regarding patient care.

   Several submodules of the Chart help manage other clinical functions. The Presenter is a unique case presentation program that displays treatment plan costs in terms of primary and secondary insurance portions and the estimated patient's portion. The Clinical Record helps you keep a comprehensive oral health evaluation for each patient. Finally, Dentrix's Perio Chart maintains and utilizes periodontal data.

Ledger

Procedures completed in the Patient Chart are automatically posted in the Ledger, where patient accounts are managed. From the Ledger, all financial transactions are recorded, including charges, payments, and adjustments. The Ledger also provides information concerning patient portion versus insurance portion, deductibles owed, and payment arrangements.

Office Manager

The Office Manager offers useful, customizable reports, including day sheets, aging reports, other financial reports, patient lists, reference reports, and others.

   The Office Manager also integrates with Microsoft Word to create effective, professional-quality letters, including welcome letters, congratulatory letters, thank you letters, a variety of appointment and continuing care (recall) reminders, progress reports, and collection notices.

Appointment List

The Appointment List displays a list of the day's appointments and provides the ability to schedule appointments and accurately track continuing care (recall) appointments, unscheduled appointments, and ASAP appointments.

Important Buttons to Know

Patient Chart

This button appears in every major toolbar throughout the Dentrix system. Choosing this button will open and display the patient's current chart. It cannot be chosen from within the Patient Chart.

xvi

Family File

This button appears in every major toolbar throughout the Dentrix system. Selecting this button will open and display the patient's current family file. It cannot be selected from within the Family File.

Ledger

This button appears in every major toolbar throughout the Dentrix system. Choosing this button will open and display the patient's current ledger. It cannot be selected from within the Ledger.

Appointments

This button appears in every major toolbar throughout the Dentrix system. Selecting this button will open the Appointment List and display the current system date. It cannot be selected from within the Appointment List.

Office Manager

This button appears in every major toolbar throughout the Dentrix system. Choosing this button will open the Office Manager. It cannot be chosen from within the Office Manager.

Select Patient

This button appears in every major toolbar throughout the Dentrix system except for the Office Manager and Appointment Book. Select this button to open a patient's Chart, Ledger, or Family File.

Quick Letters

This button appears in every major toolbar throughout the Dentrix system except the Office Manager. Quick Letters allows you to print prewritten letters concerning a patient's account or clinical diagnosis and treatment plan.

Continuing Care (Recall)

This button appears in every major toolbar throughout the Dentrix system except the Office Manager. Selecting this button allows you to quickly view recall appointments assigned to the patient and see whether an appointment has been made for each.

Office Journal

This button appears in every major toolbar throughout the Dentrix system. Acting as a contact manager, all correspondence and contact made with a patient can be tracked and recorded by clicking the Office Journal button.

Patient Questionnaire

This button appears in every major toolbar throughout the Dentrix system except the Office Manager. Selecting the Patient Questionnaire button offers access to customizable questionnaires that can be completed by patients and then stored in the Patient Questionnaire window.

Medical Alerts

This button appears in the Family File, Patient Chart, and Presenter toolbars. When a patient has a health condition requiring attention, the cross is red. Choosing this button presents a list of the patient's medical alerts. Medical alerts can also be added, edited, or deleted from this list.

Patient Picture

This button appears in all modules except the Ledger and Office Manager. Clicking this button presents a digital photograph of a patient.

Patient Alerts

This button appears in every major toolbar throughout the Dentrix system except the Office Manager. Selecting this button allows you to add or edit Patient Alerts for the selected patient.

Document Center

This button appears in every major toolbar throughout Dentrix. By clicking this button, you can view and edit documents attached to patients, providers, employers, referrals, and insurance carriers.

Patient Referrals

This button appears in every major toolbar throughout the Dentrix system except the Office Manager. It allows users to view, add, or edit patient referral information.

Introduction to Dentrix Practice Management Software

User Support

Questions regarding the use of Dentrix can be answered by referring to the Dentrix 11 User's Manual found on the software CD-ROM or by accessing the on-line help available in each Dentrix module. To access the on-line help, choose the Help option from the menu of any Dentrix module.

For questions not addressed in the user's manual or on-line help, contact Dentrix Software Support at **1-800-735-5518**.

NOTE: *The Dentrix staff is not able to assist with any hardware, network, or operating system questions or problems. Hardware, network, and operating environments vary from installation to installation; therefore, these questions should be referred to your hardware and/or operating system support representative. Operating system questions can generally be answered by reading the Windows® documentation.*

1 Orientation to the Dental Profession

INTRODUCTION

The dental profession of the 21st century will be a complex healthcare delivery system. As a member of the dental healthcare team, it is important that you understand the role of the dental assistant in all phases of the dental practice and the daily business operations. Those who will excel and become vital members of the dental healthcare team will have mastered multiple skills, will be flexible, and will work well in a team environment.

OBJECTIVES

1. List the different traits of an effective dental administrative assistant.
2. Describe the many roles of the administrative dental assistant: office manager, business manager, receptionist, insurance clerk, records manager, data processor, bookkeeper, and appointment clerk.
3. List the various members of the dental healthcare team, and discuss the roles they play in the delivery of dental care.
4. Identify the rules and function of the Health Insurance Portability and Accountability Act of 1996, Administrative Simplification, as it applies to the dental healthcare system.
5. Examine the ADA Principles of Ethics and Code of Professional Conduct, and formulate an understanding of the content by explaining, discussing, and applying the principles.

EXERCISES

1. List the personal traits of an effective dental administrative assistant.

   Be flexible and able to do more than one job at a time

   Be multiskilled to handle both dental assisting and business needs

   Be able to work in a diverse culture and maintain patient relations

   Have a strong work ethic

   Work effectively in a team environment

2. Refer to the traits you listed in question one, and select your strongest (or weakest) trait. Based on your selection, write a short paragraph (give an example) to support your selection.

   Be able to work in a diverse culture and maintain patient relations maybe a challenge or (weakness) because the different personalities and cultures are hard to cope with and understand.

3. List the responsibilities of a dental receptionist.

Projecting a positive attitude
Greeting patients
Answering the telephone
Managing income and outgoing mail
Collecting patient data

4. List the duties of a bookkeeper.

Maintaining accounts receivable records
"   " accounts payable records
Writing checks (written or electronic transfer)
Paying employees

5. Match the following job description with the appropriate administrative assistant:

a. __F__ Typically will organize and oversee the daily operations of the office staff.

b. __A__ Manages the fiscal operation of the dental practice, develops marketing campaigns, negotiates contracts, and oversees the compliance of insurance programs.

c. __D__ Maintains all aspects of the patient's clinical chart according to preset standards.

d. __C__ Responsible for entering data into the computer system.

e. __B__ Organizes and maintains the daily schedule of patients.

A. Business Manager
B. Appointment Clerk
C. Data Processor
D. Records Manager
E. Bookkeeper
F. Office Manager
G. Insurance Clerk

In the following scenarios, it will be the responsibility of the administrative dental assistant to refer the patient to a specialist. In the blank, identify the specialist you will refer the patient to for treatment.

6. Mrs. Tracy has been diagnosed with periodontal disease. Dr. Edwards instructs you to refer her to Dr. Usher for a consultation. Dr. Usher is a _Periodontics_

7. David Collins is a 4-year-old child with extensive dental caries. His mother has asked for the name of a dentist who specializes in the treatment of children. You will refer David to a _Pediatric dentistry_

8. Chris Salinas has been given the diagnosis of four impacted wisdom teeth. Dr. Edwards instructs you to refer Chris to an _Oral surgeon_

9. Judy Johnson was scheduled for an emergency visit. She has a tooth that is badly decayed. After Dr. Bradley examines Judy, he concludes that she will need a root canal. Judy will be referred to an _Endcontists_.

10. Mr. Kelly is an 85-year-old man who has been wearing <u>dentures</u> for a number of years. Because of extensive <u>alveolar bone loss on the mandibular arch</u>, Dr. Edwards would like Mr. Kelly to see a <u>Orthodontist</u> because of the complexity of the case.

11. Sally Davis is a 13-year-old young lady with very <u>crowded teeth</u>. Dr. Edwards requested a referral to an <u>Orthodontist</u> for a consultation.

12. Mrs. Gonzales was scheduled for a biopsy of oral tissue. The biopsy was sent to an <u>radiologist</u> for evaluation

13. Dr. Parker is the director and chief dentist in a government-sponsored inner city dental clinic. The specialty Dr. Parker practices is <u>dental public health</u>

14. Based on what you learned in this chapter, what do the following acronyms stand for?

D.D.S. <u>Doctor of Dental Surgery</u>

D.M.D. <u>Doctor of Medical dentistry</u>

OSHA <u>Occupational Safety and Hazard</u>

ADA <u>American Dental Association</u>

CDA <u>Certified Dental Assistant</u>

CDPMA <u>Certified Dental Practice Management Assistant</u>

ADAA <u>American Dental Assistants Association</u>

DANB <u>Dental Assisting National Board, Inc.</u>

15. List and briefly describe the five principles of ethics identified by the ADA.
1) Patent Autonomy (self-governance) 2) Non-malfeasance (do no harm) 3) Beneficence (do good) 4) Justice (fairness) 5) Veracity (truthfulness)

16. Define the following terms:
Ethics:
Category of moral judgments

Chapter **1** Orientation to the Dental Profession

Legal Standards:

Legislation regulated by boards and commission

Dental Practice Act:

Legislation that outlines the duties that can be performed by dental auxiliaries, the type of education required, and what licensure if any, is necessary for those duties

17. List and briefly describe the four sets of HIPAA standards.

Electronic Transactions and Code Sets
Privacy Rule
Security Rule   National Identifier Standard

DENTRIX EXERCISE

Before you can begin using the Dentrix software, you will need to download the CD to your computer. Please refer to the Introduction to Dentrix Practice Management Software for detailed information.

CAUTION: Please note that if you are working on a computer network, it may be necessary to change the names of the providers and the patients. You can use the same data, but the names may need to be changed to ensure that each student is creating his or her own set of providers and patients. Check with your instructor for direction.

Practice Set-Up

The version of Dentrix included with this workbook is a multiuser lockdown version. It provides access to all of the core Dentrix features but does not enable the user to change or customize practice information. Although the practice information (name, address, etc.) cannot be changed, you will be able to add information and edit settings.

Before you begin the Practice Set-up, please review the Dentrix Overview located in the Introduction to Dentrix Practice Management Software on page ix.

Starting Dentrix: Before you can begin setting up Dentrix, you must first launch the Dentrix program. You can start Dentrix in either of the following two ways:

1. Start Menu

   • Click the Windows Start button and then choose Programs. From the Programs menu, choose Dentrix. From the Dentrix menu, choose the module you wish to open. (For set-up purposes, select the Office Manager.)

2. Dentrix Quick Launch

   • The Dentrix Quick Launch icon will appear in the System Tray after Dentrix is installed. To open a module, right-click on this icon, and choose the appropriate module from the menu that appears. (For set-up purposes, select the Office Manager.)

For detailed directions, refer to the Dentrix User's Guide, Version 11, Practice Set-up: Practice Resource Set-up (page 3).

Following the direction in the User's Guide, use the following information to complete: Practice Information, Operatory Information, Provider Information, and Staff Information.

18. Practice Information. Although the practice information (name, address, etc.) cannot be changed, you will be able to add and edit settings; in addition, you will be able to add your information to administrative contact and HIPAA officer (optional).

Practice Information

Title:
Your Practice Name Here

Address:

Street
727 E Utah Valley Drive, # 500

City   ST   Zip
American Fork   UT   84003

Phone   Ext
(801)763-9300

Settings:

Administrative Contact: [   ] >>

HIPAA Officer: [   ] >>

Bank Deposit Number
1234567890

Fiscal year's beginning month (1-12): 1

○ Use Practice Info on Statements.
● Use Provider Info on Statements.

[OK]   [Cancel]

All information listed is fictitious

19. Operatory Information. Set up the following operatories:

Operatory 1

Operatory 2

Operatory 3

Operatory 4

20. Provider(s) Information. Use the following information to set up your practice providers: James Bradley, Mary Edwards, and Vivian Muensterman.

Bradley, James

Edwards, Mary A.

Muensterman, Vivian

21. Staff Information. Use the following information to set up your practice staff: Diane Blangsted, Deanna Rogers, and yourself.

Blangsted, Diane L.

Rogers, Deanna

Staff Information

	Last	First	MI
Name:	Rogers	Deanna	

ID: R152   Title:

Street
Address:

42 S Eagle Nest

City	ST	Zip
Canyon View	CA	91711

Phone: 555-4664   Ext:

SS#: 123-45-6778   [OK]   [Cancel]

Student's Information (your name and fictitious data)

Staff Information

	Last	First	MI
Name:			

ID: Title:

Street
Address:

City   ST   Zip

Phone: Ext:

SS#:   [OK]   [Cancel]

Search for the boldfaced terms in all capital letters seen in the list below in this word search puzzle.

Dental Healthcare Team Members

```
K N O I T C N U F D E D N A P X E D R C
E R N T A L H E A L T H C A R E T E E H
G A E B U S I N E S S M A N A G E R G A
M N M L E T I M B E R S T O G V L T A I
H S I W C I N N X M A Y E P B S J S N R
N Y Q T D T S A S B I G C W E Z A I A S
G S B L A B N X T U V J S Z R D Z N M I
U J B H O L F E M S R N S J M B T E E D
J V S X Y H U G M Z I A S I V A O I C E
N G R H M D C C C T F S N Q R G H G I E
Y U T Q G J D N R R N I S C A N R Y F O
N X C T T Y Z O M I S I S A E Z P H F F
A Z H L P R E D W T C X O R L C L V O T
G N D G Q Y O F R F Z O H P Y A L I H F
G D N O M G G A I D L I I X P J T E E E
T S I N O I T P E C E R M J B A D N R A
P R A C T I C E M A N A G E M E N T E K
S L V L V R E C O R D S M A N A G E R D
R E P E E K K O O B C S I J F X M B W Y
N S C C V X Q M A L O A L K L O M G G K
```

Dental **ADMINISTRATIVE** Assistant
APPOINTMENT CLERK
BOOKKEEPER
BUSINESS MANAGER
CHAIRSIDE Dental Assistant
CIRCULATING (Roving) Assistant
Certified **DENTAL ASSISTANT**

EXPANDED (Extended) **FUNCTION** Assistant
Dental **HYGIENIST**
INSURANCE CLERK
OFFICE MANAGER
Certified Dental **PRACTICE MANAGEMENT** Assistant
RECEPTIONIST
RECORDS MANAGER

2 Dental Basics

INTRODUCTION

The development of a professional dental vocabulary is essential for communicating with others. If you are unable to understand the dental language, it will be very difficult for you to carry out the fundamental duties of your job, such as appointment scheduling, insurance coding, clinical chart management, and billing.

OBJECTIVES

1. List and describe the different areas of a dental office.
2. List the basic structures of the face and oral cavity.
3. Name the basic anatomical structures and tissues of the teeth.
4. Distinguish between different numbering systems.
5. Interpret dental charting symbols.
6. Categorize basic dental procedures.
7. List basic chairside dental assisting duties, and identify OSHA and state regulations.

EXERCISES

1. Identify the different areas of the dental practice.

   a. _C_ The first area to be viewed by the patient.

   b. _d_ Area used by administrative dental assistants to perform daily business tasks.

   c. _____ A private area used to discuss confidential information with a patient.

   d. _____ Area where duties pertaining to the fiscal operation of the dental practice take place.

   e. _____ Area where patients are treated by the dentist, dental hygienist, and dental assistant.

   f. _____ Consists of a contaminated area and a clean area.

   g. _____ Dental X-rays are taken in this area.

   h. _____ Dental radiographic film is processed in this area.

   A. Sterilization area
   B. Clinical area
   C. Reception area
   D. Business office
   E. Nonclinical areas
   F. Staff room
   G. Darkroom
   H. Treatment rooms
   I. Consultation area
   J. Radiology room
   K. Storage area

2. Label the following diagram:

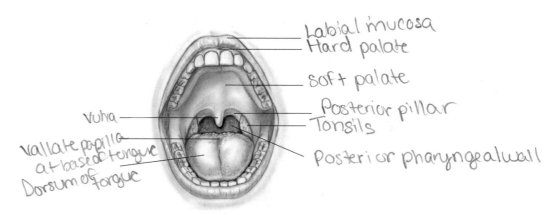

Labial mucosa
Hard palate
Soft palate
Posterior pillar
Tonsils
Posterior pharyngeal wall

Vuha
Vallate papilla at base of tongue
Dorsum of tongue

(Modified from Jarvis C: *Physical Examination & Health Assessment,* 4th ed, St. Louis, Saunders, 2004.)

3. Label the following diagram:

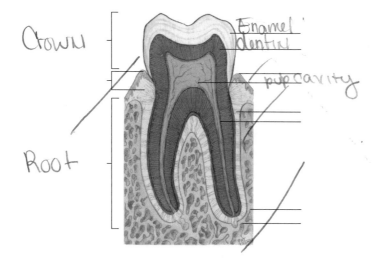

Crown
Root
Enamel
dentin
pulp cavity

(Modified from Applegate EG: *Anatomy and Physiology Learning System: Textbook,* Philadelphia, Saunders, 1995.)

Using the patient chart below, complete the following tasks:

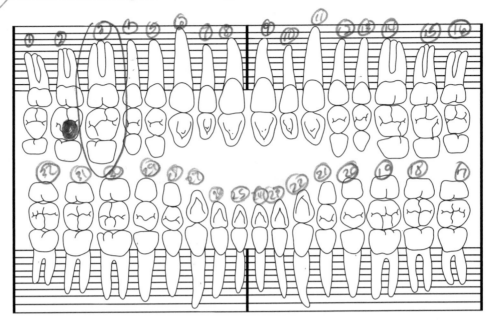

(From Weaver TK, Apfel M: *Dental Charting: Student's Manual*, Austin, Texas, Center for Occupational Curriculum Development, Division of Continuing Education, The University of Texas at Austin, 1981, p 13.)

4. Correctly number the teeth on the chart (space provided on the chart above the maxillary arch and below the mandibular arch) using the Universal Numbering System.

5. Correctly chart the following conditions using the symbols described in Chapter 2 (use red and blue pencil):
   a. Maxillary right third molar, impacted
   b. Maxillary right second molar, MO restoration
   c. Maxillary right second premolar, MOD caries
   d. Maxillary right central, bonded veneer
   e. Maxillary left central, bonded veneer
   f. Maxillary left first molar, DO restoration
   g. Maxillary left third molar, missing
   h. Mandibular left third molar, missing
   i. Mandibular left first molar, full gold crown
   j. Mandibular left cuspid, periapical abscess
   k. Mandibular right lateral, mesial composite
   l. Mandibular right second premolar, occlusal caries
   m. Mandibular right first molar, completed endodontic treatment, post and core, PFM
   n. Mandibular right third molar, needs to be extracted

DENTRIX EXERCISE

Guided Practice

Tutorial Exercise

Tutorial 1—*Select Patient:* The *Select Patient* dialog box is used throughout Dentrix. The purpose of this tutorial is to provide a comprehensive explanation of how to use all of its features.

Tutorial 4—*Patient Charting.* This tutorial will demonstrate how to chart existing, recommended, and completed procedures using the full-color Tooth Chart. Once charting is completed, it will become the database that will be used to post daily charges, print routing slips, create treatment plans, and process insurance preauthorization.

Chapter **2** **Dental Basics**

a. Open **Dentrix 11 User's Guide** (The full guide is located on the Dentrix CD that is included with the workbook.) Proceed to the Tutorial section.

b. At this time, you can print the assigned Tutorial or read from the computer screen. (NOTE: The **Dentrix 11 User's Guide** is several hundred pages long, and you will need to print only Tutorials 1 and 4. Check your computer application for the correct procedures by which to print a range of pages, or ask your instructor for directions.)

c. Switch to *Tutorial* mode

6. Complete Tutorial 1—Select Patient.

7. Complete Tutorial 4—Patient Charting.

PUZZLE

Unscramble each of the clue words. Copy the letters in the numbered cells to other cells with the same number. Solve the phrase at the bottom.

Dental Procedures

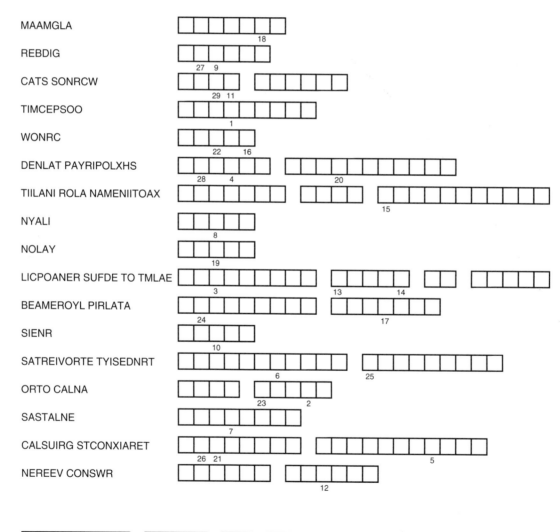

MAAMGLA

REBDIG

CATS SONRCW

TIMCEPSOO

WONRC

DENLAT PAYRIPOLXHS

TIILANI ROLA NAMENIITOAX

NYALI

NOLAY

LICPOANER SUFDE TO TMLAE

BEAMEROYL PIRLATA

SIENR

SATREIVORTE TYISEDNRT

ORTO CALNA

SASTALNE

CALSUIRG STCONXIARET

NEREEV CONSWR

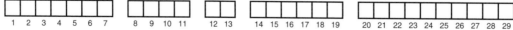

Unscramble each of the clue words. Copy the letters in the numbered cells to other cells with the same number. Solve the phrase at the bottom.

Business Letters

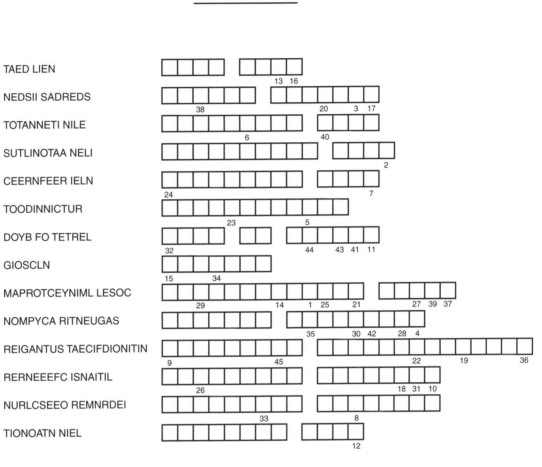

TAED LIEN

NEDSII SADREDS

TOTANNETI NILE

SUTLINOTAA NELI

CEERNFEER IELN

TOODINNICTUR

DOYB FO TETREL

GIOSCLN

MAPROTCEYNIML LESOC

NOMPYCA RITNEUGAS

REIGANTUS TAECIFDIONITIN

RERNEEEFC ISNAITIL

NURLCSEEO REMNRDEI

TIONOATN NIEL

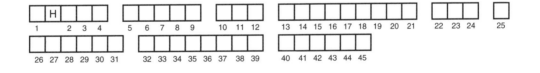

Search for the boldfaced terms in all capital letters seen in the list below in this word search puzzle.

Intergroup Communications

```
L  E  N  N  A  H  C  D  R  A  W  P  U  I  E  I  S  E  F  J  L  S  V  I  Q
P  Z  L  A  F  U  Z  N  M  A  L  P  Y  L  U  W  M  F  I  E  G  U  O  N  K
N  T  Z  O  Q  Y  M  A  A  G  J  L  E  X  P  N  I  B  N  S  V  T  X  F  L
T  M  W  A  R  T  G  O  C  D  O  C  G  J  R  E  H  N  X  H  U  A  C  O  V
U  D  A  L  Z  T  H  L  W  Y  T  B  J  J  T  Y  A  C  L  A  X  T  D  R  X
K  V  J  G  K  Z  N  Q  I  R  N  T  J  H  M  H  R  N  P  X  S  S  S  M  L
D  S  W  P  F  I  T  O  O  Y  H  W  A  X  C  G  O  J  T  K  G  D  Y  A  E
S  Z  G  G  Z  B  F  N  C  U  O  M  J  D  N  P  X  V  F  J  F  N  F  L  E
I  E  D  E  L  W  I  I  H  F  P  S  R  J  Z  D  S  C  Y  C  M  A  Y  C  H
T  R  X  U  I  C  B  X  L  L  O  A  K  Z  Z  D  V  I  K  U  L  K  T  H  J
N  O  X  X  N  F  A  F  U  T  W  N  E  J  T  A  J  J  G  H  M  N  M  A  Q
W  N  H  O  S  Q  P  B  U  N  E  N  A  W  V  C  Y  V  O  D  B  A  R  N  Y
Q  Z  I  Z  F  L  V  X  W  J  M  R  M  P  V  A  L  D  A  J  E  R  U  N  V
J  S  T  D  H  L  H  O  I  D  U  T  I  S  S  B  A  O  I  G  U  H  U  E  Q
E  S  N  I  F  I  D  H  O  R  I  Z  O  N  T  A  L  C  H  A  N  N  E  L  Z
S  R  X  P  M  L  H  C  K  V  Q  I  H  Z  G  R  C  I  H  J  D  X  T  M  O
O  E  K  K  A  I  J  X  P  P  G  W  F  E  B  Z  R  I  X  S  G  G  K  Q
O  L  O  M  G  S  N  I  J  P  K  E  L  V  Z  R  Y  K  Q  Y  P  O  V  T  F
Y  G  R  W  W  C  T  G  W  S  B  K  O  L  C  N  E  L  N  T  Q  A  U  A  F
O  O  L  G  W  S  F  P  F  X  A  K  H  E  H  E  D  O  E  Z  G  P  F  W  C
F  X  Z  L  A  C  K  O  F  T  R  U  S  T  A  S  O  W  N  V  D  H  R  G  U
C  J  C  S  F  M  N  I  D  O  Y  X  F  L  N  C  D  P  G  G  E  L  S  H  G
I  P  Y  I  D  F  B  I  W  M  O  D  Z  C  G  H  V  S  V  K  O  L  J  F  I
S  M  V  F  L  N  D  G  N  R  R  U  U  R  E  I  X  G  Z  X  D  C  B  X  Q
K  D  T  A  R  C  Y  P  U  N  T  J  H  C  Z  P  S  L  E  T  N  S  S  G  S
```

CHANGE
ELECTRONIC NOISE
FILTERING BY LEVEL
FORMAL DOWNWARD CHANNEL
HORIZONTAL CHANNEL
INFORMAL CHANNEL
LACK OF TRUST
RANK AND STATUS
Inappropriate **SPAN OF CONTROL**
TIMING
UPWARD CHANNEL
WORK OVERLOAD

JANA J. ROGERS
Medical and Dental History Information

Medical information ....Normal (not necessary to complete for this exercise)

Allergies ....Penicillin

....(enter in Med. Alert box on all appropriate forms for this patient)

Dental Information ....Normal (not necessary to complete for this exercise)

JANA J. ROGERS
Clinical Examination Information
Missing Teeth & Existing Restorations

2	MOD amalgam
13	O amalgam
14	B amalgam
18	DO amalgam
19	Sealant
30	MOD amalgam
1-16-17-32	Extracted

Soft tissue examination OK
Oral hygiene fair
Calculus moderate
Gingival bleeding none
Perio exam no

Conditions/ Treatment Indicated

3	DO amalgam
15	OB amalgam
18	B composite
30	Apical abscess/root canal
30	Core build-up (pre-fab)
30	PFM (high noble) crown

JANA J. ROGERS
Treatment Plan

Date	Tooth#	Procedure	Fee
4/12		Examination	35.00
		Prophy	60.00
		4 bite-wing x-rays	40.00
		8 PAs	16.00
5/17	3	DO amalgam	85.00
5/17	15	OB amalgam	85.00
4/24	30	Root canal	420.00
5/10	30	Post and core (pre-fab)	210.00
5/10	30	PFM (high noble)	720.00

All fees used in this exercise are for illustration only and do not represent actual fees charged for the procedures.

ANGELICA GREEN
Patient Information

Patient .... Angelica Green
Date of birth 7/20/70
If child, parent name ....
How do you wish to be addressed .... Angie
Marital status .... Married
Home address .... 724 E. Mark Ave
City .... Canyon View
State/zip .... CA 91711
Business address .... 3461 N. Cramer Ave
City .... Canyon View
State/zip .... CA 91711
Home phone 555-3004
Business phone 555-6134
Patient/parent employer .... James Tayor, DDS
Position .... RDA
How long .... 4 yrs
Spouse/parent name .... Anthony Green
Spouse employer .... Green and Associates
Position .... Accountant
How long .... 8 yrs
Who is responsible for this account .... Self
Driver's license number 60314
Method of payment .... Insurance
Purpose of call .... Toothache
Other members in this practice .... None
Whom may we thank for this referral .... Dr. Taylor
Patient/parent SS # 736-82-9176
Spouse/parent SS # 286-34-2212
Notify in case of emergency .... Grace Miller, 555-9909

Insurance Information 1st Coverage

Employee name .... Anthony Green
Employee date of birth 9-13-70
Employer .... Green and Associates
Name of Insurance Co. .... Green and Associates,
Self-Insured
Address .... 3614 E. 36th Ave
.... Canyon View 91711
Telephone 555-3615
Program or policy # .... Direct Reimbursement
Union local or group .... N/A
Social Security # 286-34-2212

Insurance Information 2nd Coverage

Employee name ....
Employee date of birth ....
Employer ....
Name of insurance co ....
Address ....
Telephone ....
Program or policy # ....
Union local or group ....
Social Security # ....
Provider .... Dr. Bradley
Privacy request .... No phone calls
First visit 3/6

ANGELICA GREEN
Medical and Dental History Information

Medical information .... Normal with following exceptions
Allergies .... Sulfa drugs and codeine
(enter in Med. Alert box on all appropriate forms for this patient)
Sensitive to latex
Bleeds easily when cut
Dental information .... Complete as much information as you can about the patient
Aware of problem .... Bleeding gums when I brush
Clench and grind teeth .... Yes
Gums bleed .... Yes

ANGELICA GREEN
Clinical Examination Information
Missing Teeth & Existing Restoration

1 .... Missing
2 .... OCC composite
3 .... B composite
14 .... DO composite
16 .... Missing
17 .... Missing
32 .... Missing

Chief Complaint: Bleeding Gums

Soft tissue examination: .... Normal
Oral hygiene: .... Good
Calculus: .... Heavy
Gingival bleeding: .... General
Perio exam: .... Yes

Conditions/Treatment Indicated

L/L .... Periodontal scaling and root planing
U/L .... Periodontal scaling and root planing
L/R .... Periodontal scaling and root planing
U/R .... Periodontal scaling and root planing

Periodontal Screening Examination

Tooth	Buccal	Lingual	Mobility	Furcation	Recession
2	676	455	1	2	1
3	876	767	1	2	1
4	444	444	0	0	0
14	876	765	1	2	1
15	453	543	1	2	1
18	547	665	1	1	0
19	767	878	1	1	0
30	455	445	1	1	0
31	667	778	1	1	0

ANGELICA GREEN
Treatment Plan

Date	Tooth #	Procedure	Fee
3/6		FMX	90.00
3/6		Comprehensive exam	45.00
4/12	L/L	Periodontal scaling & Root Plan	175.00
4/12	U/L	Periodontal scaling	175.00
4/24	L/R	Periodontal scaling & root planing	175.00
4/24	U/R	Periodontal scaling & root planing	175.00

All fees used in this exercise are for illustration only and do not represent actual fees charged for the procedures.

HOLLY BARRY
Patient Information

Patient	Holly Barry
Date of birth	3/6/28
If child, parent name	NA
How do you wish to be addressed	Mrs. Barry
Marital status	Widowed
Home address	3264 S. Vine St
City	Canyon View
State/zip	CA 91711
Business address	NA
City	
State/zip	
Home phone	555-2331
Business phone	NA
Patient/parent employer	NA
Position	NA
How long	NA
Spouse/parent name	NA
Spouse employer	NA
Position	NA
How long	NA
Who is responsible for this account	Self
Driver's license number	36788
Method of payment	Credit Card
Purpose of call	New Denture
Other members in this practice	Son
	Donald Rogers
Whom may we thank for this referral	Donald
Patient/parent SS #	111-32-4356
Spouse/parent SS #	NA
Notify in case of emergency	Donald Rogers

Insurance Information 1st Coverage

Employee name	NA
Employee date of birth	NA
Employer	NA
Name of insurance co	NA
Address	NA
Telephone	NA
Program or policy #	NA
Union local or group	NA
Social Security #	NA

Insurance Information 2nd Coverage

Employee name.. NA
Employee date of birth .... NA
Employer .... NA
Name of insurance co .... NA
Address .... NA
Telephone ....NA
Program or policy # .... NA
Union local or group ....NA
Social Security # ....NA
Provider ....Dr. Edwards
Privacy request ....none
First visit 2/4

HOLLY BARRY
Medical and Dental History Information

Medical information .... Normal (not necessary to complete for this exercise)
Allergies .... NONE (enter in Med. Alert box on all appropriate forms for this patient)
SPECIAL NOTE .... Patient cannot sit for long periods of time, must get out of the dental chair and stretch every 60 minutes
Dental information .... Normal (not necessary to complete for this exercise)

HOLLY BARRY
Clinical Examination Information
Missing Teeth & Existing Restorations

1-16 .... Missing
17-19 .... Missing
29 .... Modlb Amalgam
U ....Complete denture: Placed 1990 relined 3 times Loose fitting
L .... Partial denture: Placed 1985, broken clasp

Chief complaint: Lower right molar broken
Upper denture very loose

Soft Tissue Examination .... Normal
Oral Hygiene .... Good
Calculus ....Moderate
Gingival Bleeding ....None
Perio Exam .... Yes

Conditions/ Treatment Indicated

U .... Complete denture
29 .... PFM High noble
L .... Partial denture, metal clasp, and Framework

HOLLY BARRY
Treatment Plan

Date	Tooth #	Procedure	Fee
2/4		FMX	90.00
2/4		Examination (limited)	35.00
4/12	29	PFM	650.00
		Complete maxillary denture	950.00
4/30		Mandibular partial denture,	
		Cast metal framework	1,050.00

All fees used in this exercise are for illustration only and do not represent actual fees charged for the procedures.

43

LYNN BACCA
Patient Information

Patient .... Lynn Bacca
Date of birth 8/12/90
If child, parent name ....Chuck Bacca
How do you wish to be addressed ....Lynn
Marital status ....Child
Home address ....1812 Harman Dr.
City ....Canyon View
State/zip ....CA 91711
Business address ....34655 Vip Parkway
City .... Canyon View
State/zip ....CA 91711
Home phone 555-3421
Business phone 555-6210
Patient/parent employer ....SRVT Manufacturing
Position .... Production Manager
How long .... 8 yrs
Spouse/parent name ....Fern Bacca
Spouse employer ....Canyon View USD
Position .... Teacher
How long ....5 yrs
Who is responsible for this account .... Father
Driver's license number 878765
Method of payment ....Insurance
Purpose of call ....Exam
Other members in this practice ....Parents, Brother Steve
Whom may we thank for this referral ....Aunt, Evelyn Evatt
                                                                                       3245 S. Spring St
                                                                                       Canyon View, CA 91711
Patient/parent SS # 026-81-9217
Spouse/parent SS # 213-90-7148
Notify in case of emergency ....Parent

Insurance Information 1st Coverage

Employee name .... Chuck Bacca
Employee date of birth 7/27/65
Employer ....SRVT
Name of insurance co ....Travelers
Address .... 2111 10th Ave
                                                                                       Canyon View, CA 91711
Telephone 555-0008
Program or policy # 2345678
Union local or group 3186
Social Security # 026-81-9217

Insurance Information 2nd Coverage

Employee name .... Fern Bacca
Employee date of birth 7/5/68
Employer ....Canyon View USD
Name of insurance co .... Delta Dental of California
Address .... 99876 Hayward
                                                                                       Canyon View, CA 91711

```
Telephone ................................................................555-1098
Program or policy # ..............................................213907148
Union local or group ..............................................3216
Social Security # ..................................................213-90-7148
Provider ............................................................Dr. Bradley
Privacy request ..................................................None
First visit ........................................................4/12
```

LYNN BACCA
Medical and Dental History Information

Medical information .... Normal (not necessary to complete for this exercise)

Allergies .... (enter in Med. Alert box on all appropriate forms for this patient)

Dental information .... Normal (not necessary to complete for this exercise)

LYNN BACCA
Clinical Examination Information
Missing Teeth & Existing Restorations

No Existing Restorations or Missing Teeth

```
Soft tissue examination: ............................................. Normal
Oral hygiene: ........................................................... Good
Calculus: ................................................................. None
Gingival bleeding: ................................................... None
Perio exam: ............................................................. No
```

Conditions/ Treatment Indicated

```
3 ............................................................................ Sealant
14 .......................................................................... Sealant
19 .......................................................................... Sealant
30 .......................................................................... Sealant
```

LYNN BACCA
Treatment Plan

Date	Tooth #	Procedure	Fee
4/12		BW X-Rays (4)	40.00
		2 ANT PA's	14.00
		Prophy and Fluoride TX	54.00
4/24	3	Sealant	32.00
	14	Sealant	32.00
	19	Sealant	32.00
	30	Sealant	32.00

All fees used in this exercise are for illustration only and do not represent actual fees charged for the procedures.

DENTRIX EXERCISE

Guided Practice

Tutorial Exercise

Tutorial 2—*Entering Patient Information*. This tutorial will demonstrate how to enter a husband and wife into the Family File, using patient information available from the tutorial database. Both patients are employed, have insurance, and were referred by an existing patient. One of the family members has medical alerts and a special patient note.

Chapter **7** **Patient Clinical Records**

a. Open **Dentrix 11 User's Guide** (The full guide is located on the Dentrix CD that is included with the workbook.) Proceed to the Tutorial section.

b. At this time, you can print the assigned Tutorial or read from the computer screen. (NOTE: The **Dentrix 11 User's Guide** is several hundred pages long, and you will need to print only Tutorial 2. Check your computer application for the correct procedures by which to print a range of pages, or ask your instructor for directions.)

c. Switch to *Tutorial* mode.

13. Complete Tutorial 2—*Entering Patient Information.*

Independent Practice

Switch back to *Real Database.*

14. Prepare a Dentrix record for Jana Rogers.
   - Create a chart for the new family.
   - Add Jana as a new family member.
   - Enter insurance information.
   - Enter examination and treatment information.

15. Prepare a Dentrix record for Angelica Green.
   - Create a chart for the new family.
   - Add Angelica as a new family member.
   - Enter insurance information.
   - Enter examination and treatment information.

16. Prepare a Dentrix record for Holly Barry.
   - Create a chart for the new family.
   - Enter examination and treatment information.

17. Prepare a Dentrix record for Lynn Bacca.
   - Create a chart for the new family.
   - Add Lynn as a new family member.
   - Enter insurance information.

PUZZLE

Each letter of the alphabet has been assigned a number (e.g., O=17). Working back and forth, solve the following quote from the chapter. HINT: Look for common words (e.g., a, an, the, of).

Risk Management

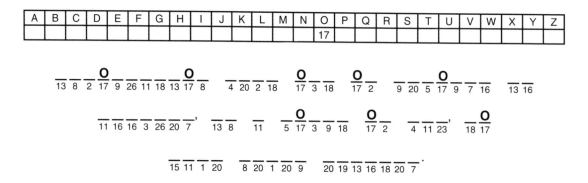

8 Information Management

INTRODUCTION

The responsibilities of the administrative dental assistant in the management of information do not end after the collection of data. These responsibilities continue, with proper storage and retrieval of information files and records. A systematic approach to filing is important to guarantee the integrity and safety of all documents.

OBJECTIVES

1. List and describe the five filing methods outlined in this chapter.
2. Classify personal names according to ARMA simplified Filing Standard Rules, by correctly indexing names as they will appear on filing labels.
3. List the types of filing methods used for filing accounts payable, accounts receivable, bank statements, financial reports, and personnel records.
4. Describe methods that can be used for filing patient information.
5. Prepare a new patient's clinical record for filing.
6. Prepare a business document for filing.

EXERCISES

1. List the five basic filing methods.

_____

_____

_____

_____

_____

_____

2. Define the following:

Indexing: _____

_____

_____

Filing unit: _____

_____

_____

Filing segment: _____

_____

_____

3. Using the personal name rule, identify which information will be placed in the following:

   Unit 1 _____

   Unit 2 _____

   Unit 3 _____

   Unit 4 _____

4. Using the business rule, identify which information will be placed in the following:

   Unit 1 _____

   Unit 2 _____

   Unit 3 _____

   Unit 4 _____

5. When a numeric filing system is used for patient's records, a key component in locating the record is:
   a. charts are arranged numerically
   b. charts are color-coded
   c. charts are randomly assigned numbers
   d. charts are cross-referenced

6. Geographic category records are filed according to:
   a. zip code
   b. area code
   c. city
   d. state
   e. all of the above

7. Subject filing is a method of filing strictly by subject. True or false, and why?

_____

_____

_____

_____

_____

8. What method indexes by date?

_____

9. **Matching:** Identify the method of filing that would be used when a system is established for the following types of business documents. If a system uses two methods, list the primary location first, and the secondary method second. For example: Personnel files are first filed by subject (primary location) and then filed alphabetically by employee (secondary method). The answer will be s/a.

a. ___/___Accounts payable

b. ___/___Accounts receivable (ledger)

c. ___/___Bank statements

d. ___/___Financial reports

e. ___/___Personnel records

f. ___/___Payroll records

g. ___/___Tax records

h. ___/___Business reports

i. ___/___Insurance reports (business)

j. ___/___Insurance claims (patient)

k. ___/___Professional correspondence

l. ___/___Patient information

S. Subject

G. Geographic

A. Alphabetical

N. Numerical

C. Chronological

10. When maintaining an active filing system it will be necessary to remove inactive records and documents. Identify two types of transfer methods, and briefly describe how each method works.

_____

_____

_____

_____

_____

_____

11. List the six basic rules for properly indexing names for filing.

_____

_____

_____

_____

_____

_____

12. For additional practice, complete Chapter 8, Critical Thinking Question 2.

_____

_____

_____

_____

ACTIVITY EXERCISE

Complete the preparation of clinical records for the following patients. Follow the guidelines listed in the text. (Anatomy of an Indexed File Folder, p. 163)

13. Jana Rogers

14. Angelica Green

15. Holly Barry

16. Lynn Bacca

Using the clues below, fill in the crossword puzzle.

Filing Methods

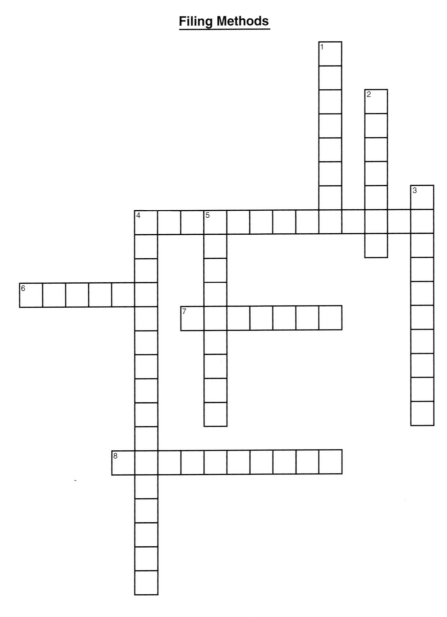

Across

4. Used to locate materials by date, month, or year
6. Used to divide filing systems into small sections
7. Filing method used for very large numbers of records
8. Categorizes records according to a location

Down

1. Arrangement of a name, subject, or number
2. Used to retrieve information according to topic
3. Follows strict rules standardized by the Association of Records Managers and Administrators
4. Identifies what other names (or name) a record is filed under
5. Used to fill the space occupied by a file that has been removed

10. Complete an appointment card for each patient.

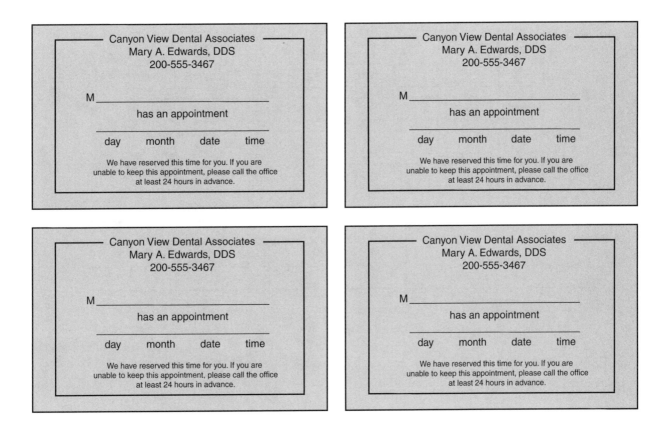

DENTRIX EXERCISE

Using the Dentrix Appointment List, matrix the appointment list using the criteria identified in Exercise 7. You will need to change the date to correspond with the current month; you may want to schedule the date 2 or 3 weeks out.

- Start Dentrix.
- Open the *Appointment List*, and click on *Set-up* and then *Practice Set-up*. Follow the steps to matrix your appointment list.
- Review the information in the Help Menu on how to enter patient information.

Independent Practice

11. Enter appointments, using the same criteria identified in Exercise 8.

PUZZLE

Rearrange the tiles to form a statement.

Scheduling

FO	TS	CA	RGE	LL	NCY	NAB	EME
O M	OF	OF	NTS	RE	TIS	DEN	ANG
REC	SHA	IR	R T	EME	IEN	PAT	D T
LE	HE	ARR	THE	IGE	BE	OBL	TS
ASO	ORD	RE	AKE				

Your task as the administrative assistant is to evaluate these concerns by identifying the problem and presenting a possible solution. You will present your findings in the form of a report at your next staff meeting.

_____

_____

_____

_____

_____

_____

_____

_____

_____

_____

_____

_____

_____

_____

DENTRIX EXERCISE (OPTIONAL)

Dentrix allows the use of multiple Continuing Care types (recall information). Review the information in the User's Guide located in the chapter, Family File, Assigning Continuing Care.

Independent Practice

7. Assign a continuing care plan for Jana Rogers, Angelica Green, Holly Barry, and Lynn Bacca.

Fit the letters in each column into the boxes directly above them to form words. Once a letter is used, cross it off. A black square indicates the end of a word. You will be able to find a completed quotation.

Recall Quotation

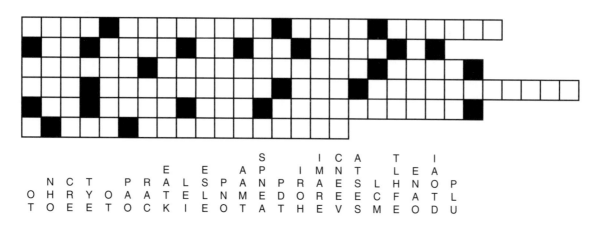

```
                              S           I     C   A     T     I
                        E     E     A     P     M   N     L     E
            N  C  T     P  R  A  L  S  P  A  N   P  R  A   S  L  H  N  O  P
            O  H  R  Y  O  A  A  T  E  L  N  M   E  D  O   R  E  C  F  A  T  L
            T  O  E  E  T  O  C  K  I  E  O  T   A  T  H   E  V  S  M  E  O  D  U
```

ADA. Dental Claim Form

HEADER INFORMATION

1. Type of Transaction (Check all applicable boxes)

☐ Statement of Actual Services   ☐ Request for Predetermination/Preauthorization

☐ EPSDT/Title XIX

2. Predetermination/Preauthorization Number

PRIMARY PAYER INFORMATION

3. Name, Address, City, State, Zip Code

OTHER COVERAGE

4. Other Dental or Medical Coverage?   ☐ No (Skip 5-11)   ☐ Yes (Complete 5-11)

5. Other Insured's Name (Last, First, Middle Initial, Suffix)

6. Date of Birth (MM/DD/CCYY)   **7. Gender** ☐ M ☐ F   **8. Subscriber Identifier (SSN or ID#)**

9. Plan/Group Number   **10. Patient's Relationship to Other Insured** (Check applicable box)   ☐ Self ☐ Spouse ☐ Dependent ☐ Other

11. Other Carrier Name, Address, City, State, Zip Code

PRIMARY INSURED INFORMATION

12. Name (Last, First, Middle Initial, Suffix), Address, City, State, Zip Code

13. Date of Birth (MM/DD/CCYY)   **14. Gender** ☐ M ☐ F   **15. Subscriber Identifier (SSN or ID#)**

16. Plan/Group Number   **17. Employer Name**

PATIENT INFORMATION

18. Relationship to Primary Insured (Check applicable box)   ☐ Self ☐ Spouse ☐ Dependent Child ☐ Other   **19. Student Status** ☐ FTS ☐ PTS

20. Name (Last, First, Middle Initial, Suffix), Address, City, State, Zip Code

21. Date of Birth (MM/DD/CCYY)   **22. Gender** ☐ M ☐ F   **23. Patient ID/Account # (Assigned by Dentist)**

RECORD OF SERVICES PROVIDED

	24. Procedure Date (MM/DD/CCYY)	25. Area of Oral Cavity	26. Tooth System	27. Tooth Number(s) or Letter(s)	28. Tooth Surface	29. Procedure Code	30. Description	31. Fee
1								
2								
3								
4								
5								
6								
7								
8								
9								
10								

MISSING TEETH INFORMATION

34. (Place an 'X' on each missing tooth)	Permanent																Primary										32. Other Fee(s)
	1	2	3	4	5	6	7	8	9	10	11	12	13	14	15	16	A	B	C	D	E	F	G	H	I	J	
	32	31	30	29	28	27	26	25	24	23	22	21	20	19	18	17	T	S	R	Q	P	O	N	M	L	K	33. Total Fee

35. Remarks

AUTHORIZATIONS

36. I have been informed of the treatment plan and associated fees. I agree to be responsible for all charges for dental services and materials not paid by my dental benefit plan, unless prohibited by law, or the treating dentist or dental practice has a contractual agreement with my plan prohibiting all or a portion of such charges. To the extent permitted by law, I consent to your use and disclosure of my protected health information to carry out payment activities in connection with this claim.

X_____
Patient/Guardian signature   Date

37. I hereby authorize and direct payment of the dental benefits otherwise payable to me, directly to the below named dentist or dental entity.

X_____
Subscriber signature   Date

BILLING DENTIST OR DENTAL ENTITY (Leave blank if dentist or dental entity is not submitting claim on behalf of the patient or insured/subscriber)

48. Name, Address, City, State, Zip Code

49. Provider ID   **50. License Number**   **51. SSN or TIN**

52. Phone Number (   )

ANCILLARY CLAIM/TREATMENT INFORMATION

38. Place of Treatment (Check applicable box)   ☐ Provider's Office ☐ Hospital ☐ ECF ☐ Other

39. Number of Enclosures (00 to 99) Radiograph(s) ☐ Oral Image(s) ☐ Model(s) ☐

40. Is Treatment for Orthodontics?   ☐ No (Skip 41-42)   ☐ Yes (Complete 41-42)

41. Date Appliance Placed (MM/DD/CCYY)

42. Months of Treatment Remaining   **43. Replacement of Prosthesis?** ☐ No ☐ Yes (Complete 44)   **44. Date Prior Placement (MM/DD/CCYY)**

45. Treatment Resulting from (Check applicable box)   ☐ Occupational illness/injury ☐ Auto accident ☐ Other accident

46. Date of Accident (MM/DD/CCYY)   **47. Auto Accident State**

TREATING DENTIST AND TREATMENT LOCATION INFORMATION

53. I hereby certify that the procedures as indicated by date are in progress (for procedures that require multiple visits) or have been completed and that the fees submitted are the actual fees I have charged and intend to collect for those procedures.

X_____
Signed (Treating Dentist)   Date

54. Provider ID   **55. License Number**

56. Address, City, State, Zip Code

57. Phone Number (   )   **58. Treating Provider Specialty**

© 2002, 2004 American Dental Association
J515 (Same as ADA Dental Claim Form – J516, J517, J518, J519)

Cat. #590154   Rev. 2-05

ADA. Dental Claim Form

HEADER INFORMATION

1. Type of Transaction (Check all applicable boxes)

- [ ] Statement of Actual Services
- [ ] Request for Predetermination / Preauthorization
- [ ] EPSDT / Title XIX

2. Predetermination / Preauthorization Number

PRIMARY PAYER INFORMATION

3. Name, Address, City, State, Zip Code

OTHER COVERAGE

4. Other Dental or Medical Coverage? [ ] No (Skip 5-11) [ ] Yes (Complete 5-11)

5. Other Insured's Name (Last, First, Middle Initial, Suffix)

6. Date of Birth (MM/DD/CCYY) | **7. Gender** [ ] M [ ] F | **8. Subscriber Identifier (SSN or ID#)**

9. Plan/Group Number | **10. Patient's Relationship to Other Insured (Check applicable box)** [ ] Self [ ] Spouse [ ] Dependent [ ] Other

11. Other Carrier Name, Address, City, State, Zip Code

PRIMARY INSURED INFORMATION

12. Name (Last, First, Middle Initial, Suffix), Address, City, State, Zip Code

13. Date of Birth (MM/DD/CCYY) | **14. Gender** [ ] M [ ] F | **15. Subscriber Identifier (SSN or ID#)**

16. Plan/Group Number | **17. Employer Name**

PATIENT INFORMATION

18. Relationship to Primary Insured (Check applicable box) [ ] Self [ ] Spouse [ ] Dependent Child [ ] Other | **19. Student Status** [ ] FTS [ ] PTS

20. Name (Last, First, Middle Initial, Suffix), Address, City, State, Zip Code

21. Date of Birth (MM/DD/CCYY) | **22. Gender** [ ] M [ ] F | **23. Patient ID/Account # (Assigned by Dentist)**

RECORD OF SERVICES PROVIDED

	24. Procedure Date (MM/DD/CCYY)	25. Area of Oral Cavity	26. Tooth System	27. Tooth Number(s) or Letter(s)	28. Tooth Surface	29. Procedure Code	30. Description	31. Fee
1								
2								
3								
4								
5								
6								
7								
8								
9								
10								

MISSING TEETH INFORMATION

34. (Place an 'X' on each missing tooth)

Permanent	Primary	32. Other Fee(s)
1 2 3 4 5 6 7 8 9 10 11 12 13 14 15 16	A B C D E F G H I J	
32 31 30 29 28 27 26 25 24 23 22 21 20 19 18 17	T S R Q P O N M L K	33. Total Fee

35. Remarks

AUTHORIZATIONS

36. I have been informed of the treatment plan and associated fees. I agree to be responsible for all charges for dental services and materials not paid by my dental benefit plan, unless prohibited by law, or the treating dentist or dental practice has a contractual agreement with my plan prohibiting all or a portion of such charges. To the extent permitted by law, I consent to your use and disclosure of my protected health information to carry out payment activities in connection with this claim.

X _____
Patient/Guardian signature   Date

37. I hereby authorize and direct payment of the dental benefits otherwise payable to me, directly to the below named dentist or dental entity.

X _____
Subscriber signature   Date

BILLING DENTIST OR DENTAL ENTITY
(Leave blank if dentist or dental entity is not submitting claim on behalf of the patient or insured/subscriber)

48. Name, Address, City, State, Zip Code

49. Provider ID | **50. License Number** | **51. SSN or TIN**

52. Phone Number (   )

ANCILLARY CLAIM/TREATMENT INFORMATION

38. Place of Treatment (Check applicable box) [ ] Provider's Office [ ] Hospital [ ] ECF [ ] Other | **39. Number of Enclosures (00 to 99)** Radiograph(s) Oral Image(s) Model(s)

40. Is Treatment for Orthodontics? [ ] No (Skip 41-42) [ ] Yes (Complete 41-42) | **41. Date Appliance Placed (MM/DD/CCYY)**

42. Months of Treatment Remaining | **43. Replacement of Prosthesis?** [ ] No [ ] Yes (Complete 44) | **44. Date Prior Placement (MM/DD/CCYY)**

45. Treatment Resulting from (Check applicable box) [ ] Occupational illness/injury [ ] Auto accident [ ] Other accident

46. Date of Accident (MM/DD/CCYY) | **47. Auto Accident State**

TREATING DENTIST AND TREATMENT LOCATION INFORMATION

53. I hereby certify that the procedures as indicated by date are in progress (for procedures that require multiple visits) or have been completed and that the fees submitted are the actual fees I have charged and intend to collect for those procedures.

X _____
Signed (Treating Dentist)   Date

54. Provider ID | **55. License Number**

56. Address, City, State, Zip Code

57. Phone Number (   ) | **58. Treating Provider Specialty**

© **2002, 2004 American Dental Association**
J515 (Same as ADA Dental Claim Form – J516, J517, J518, J519)

Cat. #590154 Rev. 2-05

25. In Tutorial Mode, complete Tutorial 5—Reviewing the Ledger.

26. In Tutorial Mode, complete Tutorial 6—Insurance Claims and Estimates.

INDEPENDENT PRACTICE

Switch back to *Real Database.*

27. Complete and print a pretreatment insurance form for Jana Rogers.

DENTRIX EXERCISE

Guided Practice

Tutorial Exercise

Tutorial 5—*Reviewing the Ledger.* This tutorial will demonstrate how to perform the common daily tasks of entering completed procedures and treatment plans, entering payments, and printing walkout statements.
Tutorial 6—*Insurance Claims.* This tutorial will demonstrate how to process primary and secondary insurance claims and pretreatment estimates.

   a. Open **Dentrix 11 User's Guide** (The full guide is located on the Dentrix CD that is included with the workbook.) Proceed to the Tutorial section.

   b. At this time, you can print the assigned Tutorial or read from the computer screen. (NOTE: The **Dentrix 11 User's Guide** is several hundred pages long, and you will need to print only Tutorials 5 and 6. Check your computer application for the correct procedures by which to print a range of pages, or ask your instructor for directions.)

   c. Switch to *Tutorial* mode.

25. Complete Tutorial 5—*Reviewing the Ledger.*

26. Complete Tutorial 6—*Insurance Claims.*

Independent Practice

Switch back to *Real Database.*

27. Complete and print a pre-treatment insurance claim form for Jana Rogers.

Find the terms listed below. The letters not used in the puzzle will spell out a phrase.

Dental Insurance Processing

```
Y T D E N T A L I N F O E G S N U R A N C E P R O C S E E S
T N S S I N G T E E V E N R O M S V V K L X W R S L E N R U
R E O F S S A D E E F I F I V Q N C F W L Y P S A Q G C V P
A M L L L F U S R E L B T F H M W N W D B L K H F X R O H E
P Y F K C H C B L L C A B E N E F I T P A Y M E N T A U P R
D A A R L H I B I A Z V Y I N S U R E D R S D P V Q H N A B
R P Z G E L A B P I E R U T A L C N E M O N R E O K C T W I
I O P D L N E I R A U D I T E W C H E W Y E O O E A D E X L
H C U I O C T O W X J J W W R O A M K F C P P C R P E R G L
T L N S N A H E C I V R E S T I F E N E B D D N T P R F N S
E G A A T T A N W F U C M S E W O K R D T E U D E Y E O I J
S E L I U E W A N U I S W U U F F T T D P X I E E O V R D E
R A O A F K U U T V N O I T A N I M R E T E D E R P O M O T
B N E P M A E T R G R U F R B F O Y N T E R E R U K C S C U
S R P O E N T E X P I R A T I O N D A T E O A F E M O Z N S
P B U N G N S E F U E O L C C U E X C X S T F K L Y T T W L
V W S S S R E E L L K R A E U N X J C E T A A M L A A X O X
A W R R O U T N E B O T S N T G E N D E R R U L E S U P D X
D T T F U B U B R F I E T S A H S Y O D A T S T N P T S T L
E T E R T T T W T O F T R U W L E B X C T S P T A U R T U X
R E R R H S N T N T L O C A U L E B F C U I O W P T R X T C
F S N O I S U L C X E L G U C O F B C F X N O X D U T I C Z
E L U R Y A D H T R I B M N D D J A B B A I J X E M T N K H
C R E B I R C S B U S C D E I E E F Y R A M O T S U C S R U
L E N A P N E P O F F E L A N L D G F F X D J P O T T U C K
F K M A E T M R H A N K Y A T T I F A F R A A O L E T R K O
N A L P Y T I N M E D N I H I F F F R N R X R S C E T E R V
O V E R C O D I N G A O N G Y M R R E R A R J L F R F R H D
B L S O D G B K B A F J T T W Y N K Y R R M A E F O F T O M
W F B S E G R A H C E L B A W O L L A I P I R R O Y F K M A
```

ADMINISTRATOR	GENDER RULE
ALLOWABLE CHARGES	INDEMNITY PLAN
AUDIT	INSURED
BALANCE BILLING	INSURER
BENEFIT PAYMENT	MANAGED CARE
BENEFIT SERVICE	NOMENCLATURE
BIRTHDAY RULE	OPEN ENROLLMENT
CAPITATION	OPEN PANEL
CLAIM	OVERBILLING
CLOSED PANEL	OVERCODING
COPAYMENT	PAYER
COVERED CHARGES	PREAUTHORIZATION
CUSTOMARY FEE	PRECERTIFICATION
DEDUCTIBLE	PREDETERMINATION
DEPENDENTS	PREFILING OF FEES
DOWNCODING	REASONABLE FEE
ENCOUNTER FORMS	SUBSCRIBER
EXCLUSIONS	SUPERBILLS
EXPIRATION DATE	THIRD PARTY
FEE FOR SERVICE	USUAL FEE
FEE SCHEDULE	

12 Inventory Management

INTRODUCTION

Ordering and managing supplies in a dental practice requires organization, communication, and the cooperation of the entire dental healthcare team. Inventory control is not limited to supplies in the clinical area. Those in the laboratory and business office must be managed as well. Tempers flare and frustration levels climb when needed supplies are not readily available. To ease tensions between team members, a systematic and well-organized inventory management system must be implemented and practiced.

OBJECTIVES

1. List the information needed to order supplies and products, and discuss how this information will be used. Define rate of use and lead time.
2. Describe the role of an inventory manager.
3. Analyze the elements of a good inventory management system, and describe how elements relate to the organization and overall effectiveness of a dental practice.
4. Compare the advantages and disadvantages of catalog ordering and supply-house services. Discuss when it is appropriate to use the two services.
5. List the information to consider before planning an order for supplies and products.
6. Describe the different sections of a Material Safety Data Sheet, and discuss what information is important to an inventory manager.

EXERCISES

1. List the information needed for ordering supplies.

_____

_____

_____

_____

_____

_____

_____

_____

73

2. List five responsibilities of an inventory manager.

_____

_____

_____

_____

_____

3. Define rate of use.

_____

_____

_____

4. Define lead time.

_____

_____

_____

5. Define back order.

_____

_____

_____

6. A good inventory management system involves seven elements. List two elements and describe how they relate to the organization of an effective dental practice.

_____

_____

_____

_____

_____

74

Using the scenarios below, determine whether to use a supply house or a catalog to order supplies. Identify which method you will use, and explain why.

7. You have recently been hired as the new inventory manager for a large dental practice. After looking in the storage area, you realize you don't recognize some of the products.

_____

_____

_____

_____

_____

8. The dentist informs you that he has hired a new hygienist and wants to send out a mass mailing within the week publicizing her addition to the dental healthcare team. You will print the postcards in the office. When you check the inventory, you realize that you do not have enough postcards.

_____

_____

_____

_____

Use the MSDS sheet for Ultra-Etch 35% (Anatomy of an MSDS, Chapter 12) to answer the following questions.

9. What is the chemical name for Ultra-Etch 35%?

_____

10. What physical state does the product have?
    a. gas
    b. liquid
    c. solid
    d. other

11. True/false: The product carries an odor. _____

12. If the product catches fire, how would you put it out?

_____

13. Is the product incompatible with another substance? If yes which one(s)?

_____

14. If the product comes in contact with your eyes, will it damage them?_____

_____

15. How would you protect your eyes when using this product?

_____

16. How should you dispose of the product?

_____

17. Who prepared this MSDS sheet?

_____

PUZZLE

Search for the terms in this word search puzzle.

Inventory Management

```
E  G  N  I  S  A  H  C  R  U  P  L  W  U  H
Y  L  U  M  H  E  X  P  E  N  D  A  B  L  E
R  E  B  S  T  C  U  D  O  R  P  F  J  L  F
O  A  O  A  E  R  T  J  R  R  V  F  B  U  I
T  D  F  E  M  Q  E  A  D  I  M  A  M  Q  L
N  T  M  R  C  U  U  D  E  E  S  Z  S  W  F
E  I  N  A  A  P  S  I  R  O  D  N  E  V  L
V  M  R  E  T  U  R  N  P  O  L  I  C  Y  E
N  E  E  G  A  M  Z  S  O  M  K  D  H  N  H
I  M  X  A  L  S  I  H  I  C  E  C  X  O  S
O  E  B  R  O  D  A  N  N  K  N  N  A  B  E
A  G  T  O  G  S  P  I  T  Q  X  O  T  B  J
K  R  A  T  E  O  F  U  S  E  M  J  N  I  T
E  M  E  S  U  O  H  Y  L  P  P  U  S  U  J
S  E  I  L  P  P  U  S  K  S  N  G  D  U  Q
```

BACK ORDER	OSHA
CATALOG	PRODUCTS
CONSUMABLE	PURCHASING
DISPOSABLE	RATE OF USE
EQUIPMENT	REORDER POINTS
EXPENDABLE	RETURN POLICY
INVENTORY	SHELF LIFE
LEAD TIME	STORAGE AREAS
MSDS	SUPPLIES
NONCONSUMABLE	SUPPY HOUSE
ORDER	VENDOR

13 Financial Arrangements and Collection Procedures

INTRODUCTION

The responsibility for collecting fees is shared by all members of the dental healthcare team. The team will establish the policies and then follow them. The administrative dental assistant has the most visible task. After a treatment plan is drawn up, the administrative dental assistant will write the financial plan, present the plan to the patient, and then monitor compliance with the plan. If the plan is not followed, it is usually the administrative dental assistant who initiates collection procedures.

OBJECTIVES

1. List the elements of a financial policy, and discuss the qualifying factors for each of the elements.
2. Describe the different types of financial plans, and explain how they can be applied in a dental practice.
3. State the purpose of managing accounts receivable. Describe the role of the administrative dental assistant in managing accounts receivable.
4. Classify the different levels of the collection process.
5. Place a telephone collection call.
6. Process a collection letter.
7. Interpret aging reports and implement proper collection procedures.

EXERCISES

1. Match the payment plan to its definition.

   a. _____ Payment is spread out over time

   b. _____ Payment is paid by third party carrier

   c. _____ Payment installments are paid directly to the dental practice

   d. _____ Payment is divided by length of treatment

   e. _____ Another form of payment in full. Payment amount will be discounted and deposited directly into the practice's account

   f. _____ Payment is made immediately after dental visit by patient

   g. _____ Payment installments directed by a loan company

   A. Insurance billing
   B. Payment in full
   C. Outside payment plan
   D. In-house payment plan
   E. Extended payment plan
   F. Divided payment plan
   G. Credit card
   H. Creative payment plan

2. List the six steps to be followed in placing a telephone collection call.

_____

_____

_____

_____

_____

_____

3. At what level in the collection process should a letter be written?
   a. Level one
   b. Level two
   c. Level three
   d. Level four
   e. Level five

4. List at least two requirements of a properly written collection letter.

_____

_____

5. Match the following time intervals with the level of the collection process.

   a. _____ 0-30 days   A. Telephone reminder
   b. _____ 30-60 days   B. Ultimatum
   c. _____ 60-90 days   C. Mailed reminder
   d. _____ 90-120 days   D. Statement
   e. _____ Longer than 120 days   E. Collection letter
   f. _____ No response to letter   F. Turning of account over to collection
                                           G. Friendly reminder

ACTIVITY EXERCISES

Use information located on the Treatment Plan for each of the following patients to complete a Financial Arrangement Form (located at the back of the workbook).

Jana Rogers   Angelica Green
Holly Barry   Lynn Bacca

Jana Rogers

Jana's parents both have dental insurance. After their combined benefits are calculated, it has been determined that the total benefits paid will be $1,200.00.

As the Administrative Dental Assistant, you propose the following financial arrangements.
   Initial payment .... $ 75.00
   Insurance estimated payment $1,200.00
   The balance is to be paid in 3 monthly payments.
Use the completed Financial Arrangement forms to answer the following questions.

6. What is the total estimate of treatment? $_____

7. What is the balance of the estimate due? $_____

8. What is the monthly payment? $_____

Angelica Green

Angelica is covered by a direct reimbursement plan. Her plan will pay 60% of the total estimate of treatment. In addition, Dr. Edwards will give Angelica a 10% professional courtesy discount on the balance after the insurance estimate. It is agreed that Angelica will pay the balance in six monthly payments.

Complete a Financial Arrangement Form for Angelica, and use the information to answer the following questions:

9. What is the total estimate of treatment? $_____

10. What is the insurance estimate? $_____

11. What is the amount of the discount? $_____

12. What is the balance of the estimate due? $_____

13. What is the monthly payment? $_____

Holly Barry

Mrs. Barry is a senior citizen and will receive a 12% Senior Citizen Discount. She has made arrangements to pay the balance in full (credit card) on April 12.

Complete a Financial Arrangement form for Mrs. Barry and use the information to answer the following questions.

14. What is the total estimate of treatment? $_____

15. What is the amount of the discount? $_____

16. What is the balance of estimate due? $_____

Lynn Bacca

Lynn's parents both have dental insurance. The combined payment will be 100% of the total estimate for treatment, less a $50.00 deductible.

Complete a Financial Arrangement Form for Lynn, and use the information to answer the following questions:

17. What is the total estimate of treatment? $_____

18. What is the insurance estimate? $_____

DENTRIX EXERCISE (OPTIONAL)

Using the Dentrix software, you will be able to present treatment plans and set up financial arrangements. For this exercise, read the information in the User's Guide that is located in the chapter, *Patient Chart, Treatment Plan Presenter and Ledger, Setting Up Financial Arrangements.*

Independent Practice

Use the information in the *Activity Exercises* to complete a treatment plan and set up financial arrangements for a patient (you can select Jana, Holly, Angelica, or Lynn).

PUZZLE

Each letter of the alphabet has been assigned a number (e.g., E=1). Working back and forth, solve the following quote from the chapter. HINT: Look for common words (e.g., a, an, the, of).

Financial Arrangements

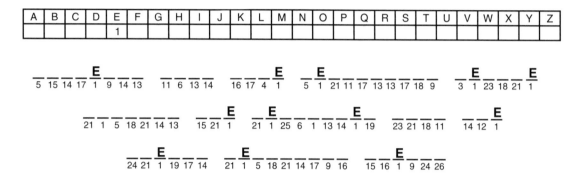

A	B	C	D	E	F	G	H	I	J	K	L	M	N	O	P	Q	R	S	T	U	V	W	X	Y	Z
				1																					

```
_ _ _ _ E _ _ _     _ _ _ _     _ _ _ E     E _ _ _ _ _ _ _ _     _ E _ _ E
5 15 14 17 1 9 14 13   11 6 13 14   16 17 4 1   5 1 21 11 17 13 13 17 18 9   3 1 23 18 21 1

_ _ _ _ _ _ _     _ _ E     E _ _ _ _ E _ _ _     _ _ _ _     _ _ E
21 1 5 18 21 14 13   15 21 1   21 1 25 6 1 13 14 1 19   23 21 18 11   14 12 1

_ _ E _ _ _     _ E _ _ _ _ _ _ _     _ _ E _ _ _
24 21 1 19 17 14   21 1 5 18 21 14 17 9 16   15 16 1 9 24 26
```

80

Chapter **13** **Financial Arrangements and Collection Procedures**

7. Proof of posting

Column D total .... $_____

Plus Column A total .... $_____

Sub total .... $_____

Less Columns B1 & B2 .... $_____

Must equal Column C .... $_____

8. Accounts receivable control

Previous day's total .... $ 1,098.10

Plus Column A total .... $_____

Sub total .... $_____

Less Columns B1 & B2 .... $_____

Total accounts receivable .... $_____

9. Accounts receivable proof

Accts receivable 1st of month .... $ 0000.00

Plus Column A month to date .... $_____

Sub total .... $_____

Less Columns B1 & B2 mo to date .... $_____

Total accounts receivable .... $_____

DAILY LOG OF CHARGES AND RECEIPTS

DATE __4/12__   SHEET NUMBER _____   A   B1   B2   C   D

	DATE	FAMILY MEMBER	PROFESSIONAL SERVICES	CHARGE		CREDITS PYMTS.	CREDITS ADJ	NEW BALANCE	PREVIOUS BALANCE	NAME
1	4/12	Rose	ins. pmt./adj.			98 00	12 00	80 00	190 00	Rose Budd
2	4/12	Frank	NSF	80 00		—	—	80 00	0	Frank Williams
3	4/12	Judy	payment	—		62 00	—	<22 00>	40 00	Judy Coulson
4	4/12	Dawn	Restorative	230 00		0	—	240 00	10 00	Dawn Johnson
5	4/12	Maria	prophy/c.pmt.	62 00		62 00	—	0	0	Marie Gonzales
6	4/12	Angela	FMX	80 00		62 00	—	80 00	62 00	Angela Brown
7	4/12	Mark	Composite	246 00		—	24 60	221 40	0	Mark Vail
8	4/12	Lois	ins. pmt.	—		630 00	20 00	171 00	821 00	Lois Tracy
9										
10										
11										
12										
13										
14										
15										
16										
17										
18										
19										
20										
21										
22										
23										
24										
25										
26										
27										
28										
29										
30										
31										
32										

TOTALS — THIS PAGE ▶
TOTALS — PREVIOUS PAGE ▶ | 3240 00 | 2163 00 | <21 10> | 5419 10 | 4321 00
TOTALS — MONTH-TO-DATE ▶

Col. "A"   Col. "B-1"   Col. "B-2"   Col. "C"   Col. "D"

Scenario: As part of your daily routine, you will print out a copy of the appointment list for each operatory and a routing slip for the patients you have scheduled for April 12 (Jana Rogers, Angelica Green, Holly Barry and Lynn Bacca). Organize your patients' clinical records and appropriate printouts in preparation for the day. At the end of each patient's appointment, you will post all transactions and print out insurance claims and walkout statements (you will complete the daily routine during the Chapter 17 exercise).

You can print the ***routing slips*** and ***appointment list*** from the ***Dentrix Office Manager*** mode. From the tool bar, click ***Reports***, select ***Lists***, then ***Daily***.

Posting Transactions (Review Tutorial #5, and use ***Help*** for detailed instructions.)

Independent Practice

Use the information that you have already completed in previous exercises (Chapter 13, Activity Exercises 6-18, and Chapter 14, Posting information). Note: For this exercise, the previous balance for each patient is zero.

At the end of the exercise, you will have printed the following:

10. Appointment list for each operatory
11. Routing slip for Jana, Angelica, Holly and Lynn
12. Walkout statement for each patient
13. Insurance form for Jana and Lynn

Optional Exercise

For added practice, you can post all transactions for each of the four patients (see Workbook Chapter 7 for treatment plan details).

Search for the terms in this word search puzzle.

Bookkeeping Terms

```
L  A  K  W  R  H  I  E  A  Q  T  M  H  I  D  P  K  E  S  G
C  S  L  S  P  E  O  C  Z  Y  Q  P  O  J  R  J  L  O  N  J
C  Y  C  L  P  G  C  O  A  A  N  Q  V  O  D  B  O  I  J  F
Q  L  Z  V  S  I  T  E  G  V  K  R  O  W  A  R  T  P  R  B
O  I  R  C  A  K  L  A  I  U  K  F  Y  V  N  N  N  E  Y  L
T  W  H  R  P  C  V  S  N  P  O  Y  I  H  U  D  E  G  E  W
U  M  X  Y  X  H  C  Y  G  F  T  E  L  O  T  V  K  B  K  L
N  J  R  H  E  Z  G  O  P  N  C  S  C  L  G  O  P  O  Q  G
Y  F  J  Q  N  R  B  O  U  E  I  C  T  T  O  W  B  A  S  G
C  I  V  J  P  M  S  P  R  N  A  T  K  L  G  O  B  R  G  N
Y  N  J  D  D  T  O  S  Q  N  T  T  U  T  D  W  I  D  H  I
B  Y  S  N  I  S  T  F  R  S  Y  S  G  O  H  Q  Y  S  A  P
A  F  I  N  A  N  C  I  A  L  R  E  P  O  R  T  S  Y  T  E
B  Q  G  K  U  G  D  A  T  T  V  K  N  A  B  K  G  S  H  E
C  T  L  O  N  D  J  P  M  M  A  S  B  D  Y  J  E  T  H  K
S  Y  C  T  X  X  H  C  D  X  M  F  U  C  V  A  Q  E  N  K
F  C  T  H  O  M  B  A  J  G  M  F  W  P  B  S  B  M  R  O
A  N  N  X  S  C  C  H  A  R  G  E  S  L  I  P  E  L  C  O
L  A  N  R  U  O  J  Y  L  I  A  D  Z  A  M  G  S  K  E  B
S  U  T  S  Y  T  X  C  H  H  A  Z  G  B  Y  O  M  K  W  E
```

ACCOUNTING	DAILY JOURNAL
ACCOUNTS PAYABLE	FINANCIAL REPORTS
ACCOUNTS RECEIVABLE	PEGBOARD SYSTEM
AGING	PROOF OF POSTING
BOOKKEEPING	RECEIPTS
CHARGE SLIP	ROUTING SLIPS

16 Office Equipment

INTRODUCTION

Office equipment helps the administrative dental assistant organize and perform tasks and save time by integrating different types of procedures. Equipment is selected on the basis of the needs of the staff. Equipment can be divided into two broad categories: equipment used to gather, transfer, and store information; and equipment used to create a working environment that is safe, organized, and functional.

OBJECTIVES

1. List the components of a dental practice information system, and explain the function of each component.
2. Categorize the different functions of a dental practice telecommunication system.
3. Describe the features of a telephone system, and explain how they can be used in a modern dental practice.
4. Design an ergonomic workstation. Identify important elements, and state their purpose.

EXERCISES

1. List and define the components of a dental practice information system.

_____

_____

_____

_____

_____

2. List the features of a telephone system.

_____

_____

_____

_____

_____

_____

_____

_____

_____

_____

3. List the functions of a telecommunication system, and describe how it can be used in a dental practice.

_____

_____

_____

_____

_____

4. List seven factors to consider when setting up an ergonomic workstation.

_____

_____

_____

_____

_____

_____

_____

_____

_____

5. Match the following terms to their definitions:

a. _____ Peripheral device used to activate   A. CPU
              commands   B. Keyboard
b. _____ Similar to a television screen   C. Mouse
c. _____ Information needed for the computer to   D. Scanner
              be able to function   E. Modem
d. _____ Used to back up information   F. Monitor
e. _____ Main operating component of hardware   G. Printer
f. _____ Digitizes information from a document   H. Storage device
g. _____ Produces a hard copy of information   I. Operating system
h. _____ Most common input device
i. _____ Transfers information

6. Define intraoffice communications.

_____

7. List the different types of intraoffice communication systems.

_____

_____

_____

_____

_____

_____

_____

          Chapter **16** **Office Equipment**

8. List the types of office machines found in a dental practice.

_____

_____

_____

_____

_____

Define the following terms:

9. Ergonomics _____

10. Background noise _____

11. Lighting _____

Ergonomic Problem Solving

12. Sally, the administrative dental assistant, is complaining of lower back pain. What should she check on her chair to rectify this problem?

_____

_____

_____

_____

13. Kevin, the business manager, is complaining of eyestrain. What can he do with his video display terminal to help alleviate the strain?

_____

_____

_____

_____

_____

100

14. Hope, the insurance clerk, has been given a diagnosis of carpal tunnel syndrome. What can she do with her keyboard and mouse to help reduce the strain?

_____

_____

_____

_____

_____

PUZZLE

Unscramble each of the clue words. Copy the letters in the numbered cells to other cells with the same number to spell out a phrase.

Ergonomics

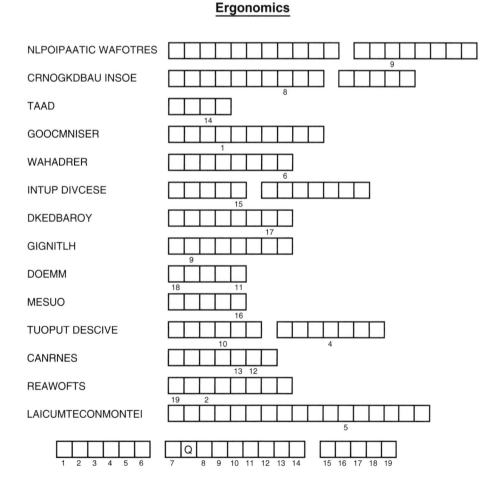

NLPOIPAATIC WAFOTRES

CRNOGKDBAU INSOE

TAAD

GOOCMNISER

WAHADRER

INTUP DIVCESE

DKEDBAROY

GIGNITLH

DOEMM

MESUO

TUOPUT DESCIVE

CANRNES

REAWOFTS

LAICUMTECONMONTEI

17 Computerized Dental Practice

INTRODUCTION

The use of computers in a dental practice is becoming standard. Computers help staff members to manage office functions, submit insurance claims, track patients, schedule appointments, and record treatments. It will be the duty of an administrative dental assistant to become familiar with and be capable of using a computer system.

OBJECTIVES

1. Compare the three levels of function of dental practice management software, and discuss the applications.
2. List the functions to consider when selecting dental practice management software.
3. Discuss the role of the administrative dental assistant in the operation of a computerized dental practice.
4. Identify the different computer tasks performed by the administrative dental assistant.
5. Compare the daily routines for which a computer system and a manual system may be used, and discuss the differences and similarities of these types of systems.
6. Describe the importance of a computer system back-up routine.

EXERCISES

1. Briefly describe the three levels of function of dental practice management software.

   Level One, Basic Systems:

   _____

   _____

   _____

   Level Two, Intermediate Systems:

   _____

   _____

   _____

   Level Three, Advanced Systems:

   _____

   _____

   _____

2. Identify the level of the dental practice management software at which the following functions can be performed (there may be more than one level):

Function	Basic	Intermediate	Advanced
A. Word processing	_____	_____	_____
B. Electronic scheduling	_____	_____	_____
C. Retain demographic information	_____	_____	_____
D. Maintain clinical information	_____	_____	_____
E. Provide software security	_____	_____	_____
F. Process insurance information	_____	_____	_____
G. Personalize recall procedures	_____	_____	_____
H. Digital radiographs	_____	_____	_____

3. List the functions you should consider when selecting dental management practice software.

_____

_____

_____

_____

_____

_____

_____

_____

_____

_____

4. Describe at least two reasons why dental practice management software is important to a dental practice.

_____

_____

104

Describe the functions of the management practice software package that are of use to each of the following members of the dental healthcare team:

5. Accountant: _____

6. Hygienist: _____

7. Administrative dental assistant: _____

8. Insurance clerk: _____

9. Describe the role of the administrative dental assistant in the operation of a computerized dental practice.

_____

_____

_____

_____

_____

_____

10. What are the advantages of using a computerized system?

_____

_____

_____

_____

_____

_____

11. List the daily procedures performed with the use of computerized dental software.

_____

_____

_____

_____

_____

_____

12. Describe the importance of backing up a computerized dental practice system.

_____

_____

_____

_____

_____

13. Match the following computerized dental software terms to their definitions:

a. _____ Appears when additional information is needed

b. _____ Identifies software being used

c. _____ Provides information about current screen

d. _____ Arranges parts of screens in logical order

e. _____ Icons and buttons that identify commonly used features

f. _____ Identifies name of user

g. _____ Provides quick access to selected features

A. Menu Bar
B. Power Bar
C. Status Bar
D. Status Window
E. Tabbed Screen
F. Title Bar
G. Toolbar

DENTRIX EXERCISE

Guided Practice

Tutorial Exercise

Tutorial 7—*Printing Reports*. This tutorial demonstrates how to generate, select, and print individual and batch reports.

Tutorial 8—*Daily Routines*. The preceding tutorials have demonstrated several routine tasks that can be accomplished with the use of Dentrix. This tutorial will cover two additional suggested daily routines: printing the day sheet (charges and receipts) and following daily back-up procedures.

a. Open **Dentrix 11 User's Guide** (The full guide is located on the Dentrix CD that is included with the workbook.) Proceed to the Tutorial section.

b. At this time, you can print the assigned Tutorial or read from the computer screen. (Note: The **Dentrix 11 User's Guide** is several hundred pages long, and you will need to print only Tutorials 7 and 8. Check your computer application for the correct procedures by which to print a range of pages, or ask your instructor for directions.)

c. Switch to *Tutorial* mode.

14. Complete Tutorial 7—Printing Reports.

15. Complete Tutorial 8—Daily Routines.

Independent Practice

Switch back to *Real Database*.

Scenario: You have just completed all of the data entry for the day (this is the conclusion of the exercise you started in Chapters 13 and 14), and you are ready to complete the end-of-day routine.

16. Print the day sheet.
    - Chronologically
    - Alphabetically
    - By provider

17. Print deposit slips.

PUZZLE

Unscramble each of the clue words. Take the letters that appear in the circle boxes and unscramble them for the final message.

Computerized Dental Practice

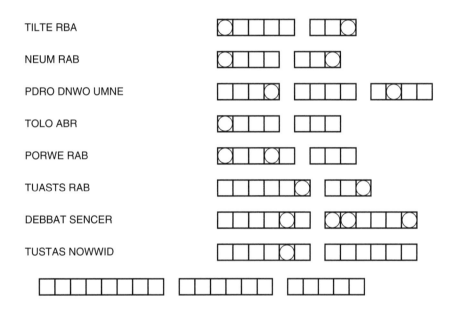

TILTE RBA

NEUM RAB

PDRO DNWO UMNE

TOLO ABR

PORWE RAB

TUASTS RAB

DEBBAT SENCER

TUSTAS NOWWID

Appendix: Forms Needed

(All forms in this section courtesy of the Dental Record, Wisconsin Dental Association, Milwaukee, WI.)

Jana Rogers

© 2003 Wisconsin Dental Association
(800) 243-4675

welcome

| | | | | | |
PATIENT NUMBER

Date _____

Patient's Name _____   Date of Birth _____ ❑ Male ❑ Female
Last   First   Initial

If Child: Parent's Name _____

How do you wish to be addressed _____
Single ❑   Married ❑   Separated ❑   Divorced ❑   Widowed ❑   Minor ❑

Residence - Street _____

City _____ State _____ Zip _____

Business Address _____

Telephone: Res. _____ Bus. _____

Fax _____ Cell Phone # _____

eMail _____

Patient/Parent Employed By _____

Present Position _____

How Long Held _____

Spouse/Parent Name _____

Spouse Employed By _____

Present Position _____

How Long Held _____

Who is Responsible for this account _____

Drivers License No. _____

Method of Payment: Insurance ❑   Cash ❑   Credit Card ❑

Purpose of Call _____

Other Family Members in this Practice _____

_____

Whom may we thank for this referral _____

Patient/parent Social Security No. _____

Spouse/Parent Social Security No. _____

Someone to notify in case of emergency not living with you _____

_____

DENTAL INSURANCE 1ST COVERAGE

Employee Name _____ Date of Birth _____
Employer Name _____ Yrs. _____
Name of Insurance Co. _____
Address _____

_____

Telephone _____
Program or policy # _____
Social Security No. _____
Union Local or Group _____

DENTAL INSURANCE 2ND COVERAGE

Employee Name _____ Date of Birth _____
Employer Name _____ Yrs. _____
Name of Insurance Co. _____
Address _____

_____

Telephone _____
Program or policy # _____
Social Security No. _____
Union Local or Group _____

CONSENT:
I consent to the diagnostic procedures and treatment by the dentist necessary for proper dental care.

I consent to the dentist's use and disclosure of my records (or my child's records) to carry out treatment, to obtain payment, and for those activities and health care operations that are related to treatment or payment.

I consent to the disclosure of my records (or my child's records) to the following persons who are involved in my care (or my child's care) or payment for that care.

_____

My consent to disclosure of records shall be effective until I revoke it in writing.

I authorize payment directly to the dentist or dental group of insurance benefits otherwise payable to me. I understand that my dental care insurance carrier or payor of my dental benefits may pay less than the actual bill for services, and that I am financially responsible for payment in full of all accounts. By signing this statement, I revoke all previous agreements to the contrary and agree to be responsible for payment of services not paid, by my dental care payor.

I attest to the accuracy of the information on this page.

PATIENT'S OR GUARDIAN'S SIGNATURE

_____

DATE _____

Form No. T110R

REGISTRATION

Jana Rogers

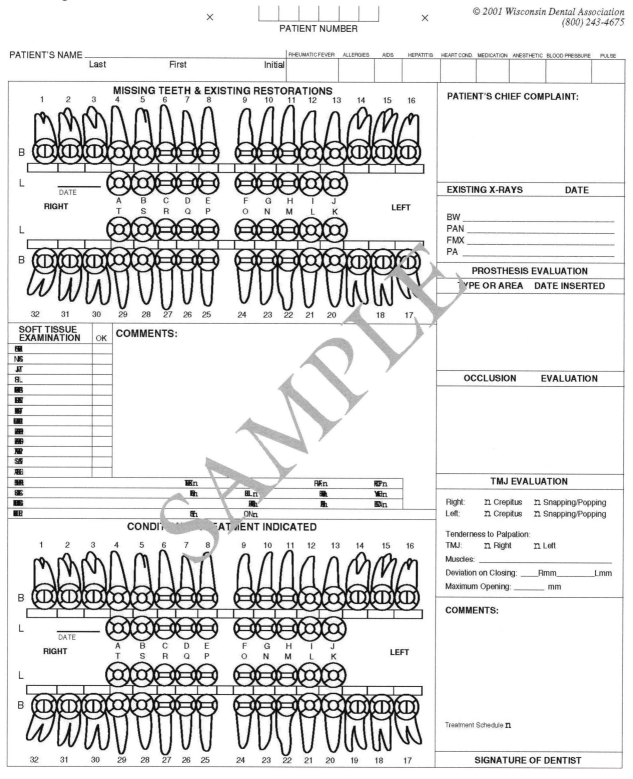

×   PATIENT NUMBER   ×

PATIENT'S NAME _____
Last   First   Initial

RHEUMATIC FEVER | ALLERGIES | AIDS | HEPATITIS | HEART COND. | MEDICATION | ANESTHETIC | BLOOD PRESSURE | PULSE

MISSING TEETH & EXISTING RESTORATIONS

1 2 3 4 5 6 7 8 9 10 11 12 13 14 15 16

B

L

DATE

RIGHT   A B C D E   F G H I J   LEFT
   T S R Q P   O N M L K

L

B

32 31 30 29 28 27 26 25   24 23 22 21 20   18 17

PATIENT'S CHIEF COMPLAINT:

EXISTING X-RAYS   **DATE**

BW _____
PAN _____
FMX _____
PA _____

PROSTHESIS EVALUATION
TYPE OR AREA   DATE INSERTED

OCCLUSION   **EVALUATION**

SOFT TISSUE EXAMINATION	OK

COMMENTS:

TMJ EVALUATION

Right: ⊓ Crepitus   ⊓ Snapping/Popping
Left: ⊓ Crepitus   ⊓ Snapping/Popping

Tenderness to Palpation:
TMJ: ⊓ Right   ⊓ Left
Muscles: _____
Deviation on Closing: ____Rmm _____Lmm
Maximum Opening: _____ mm

COMMENTS:

CONDITIONS & TREATMENT INDICATED

1 2 3 4 5 6 7 8 9 10 11 12 13 14 15 16

B

L

DATE

RIGHT   A B C D E   F G H I J   LEFT
   T S R Q P   O N M L K

L

B

32 31 30 29 28 27 26 25   24 23 22 21 20 19 18 17

Treatment Schedule ⊓

SIGNATURE OF DENTIST

Form No. T170CE

CLINICAL EXAMINATION

115

Appendix

Jana Rogers

PATIENT NUMBER

© 2001 Wisconsin Dental Association
(800) 243-4675

PATIENT'S NAME _____

	Last	First	Initial	Date

DATE	TREATMENT PLAN	FEE	ALTERNATE TREATMENT	FEE	PROB # ASGN

SAMPLE

RELEASE:

I accept the above treatment plan. I understand that because of unexpected circumstances, the treatment, the fees for treatment and/or the materials required as explained to me at this time, may require some changes after actual care has begun.

PATIENT'S/GUARDIAN'S SIGNATURE _____ DATE _____

ANEST.		MED. ALERT

Form No. T201TP

TREATMENT PLAN

Jana Rogers × 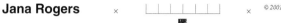 × © 2001 Wisconsin Dental Association
(800) 243-4675

PATIENT'S NAME_____

Last	First	Initial

AGREEMENT TO PAY FOR DENTAL SERVICES

Agreement to Pay. For services rendered or to be rendered to me, or to others at my request, I promise to pay to Dentist $_____, plus interest and other charges as stated below ("Obligations"). I will make the payments described in the payment schedule to Dentist at the address shown on the opposite side of this form.

Federally Required Disclosures. The calculations shown below are computed on the assumption that each payment will be made in full on the date due:

ITEMIZATION OF AMOUNT FINANCED

Dental Fees   Down Payment   Amount Financed

$ _____ − $ _____ = $ _____

ANNUAL PERCENTAGE RATE The cost of your credit as a yearly rate. _____%	FINANCE CHARGE The dollar amount the credit will cost you. $_____	Amount Financed The amount of credit provided to you or on your behalf. $_____	Total of Payments The amount you will have paid after you have made all payments as scheduled. $_____	Total Sale Price The total cost of your purchase on credit, including your downpayment of $_____ $_____

Your payment schedule will be: _____ equal consecutive installments of $_____ each, and one final installment of _____ on the _____ day of each successive month beginning_____ , 19_____.

  Late Charge. If a payment is not paid on or before the 10th day after the due date, I may be charged $10.00 or 5.00% of the unpaid amount, whichever is less.
  If I pay off early, I will not have to pay a penalty, and I may be entitled to a refund of unearned finance charges.
  See your contract documents for any additional information about nonpayments, default, any required repayment in full before the scheduled date, and prepayment refunds and penalties.

Other Charges. I agree to pay a charge of _____ for each check presented for payment and returned unpaid. I also agree to pay all costs of collection, to the extent not prohibited under law.

Application of Payments. Unless otherwise required by applicable law, payments will be applied as directed by Dentist.

Default and Remedies. I will be in default of my Obligations under this Agreement if I have an amount outstanding which exceeds one full payment which has remained unpaid for more than 10 days after the scheduled or deferred due dates; or the first or last payment is not paid within 40 days of its due date.

In the event of default, the Dentist shall:
  A. Have all the rights and remedies provided by law and this Agreement. All remedies shall be cumulative and ___ the exercise of one shall not prevent the exercise of any other remedies.
  B. Upon default the Dentist may, at its option, accelerate the amount due, without notice. In that event, the Obligations shall become payable after notice is provided and the right to cure has expired.

Miscellaneous.
  A. To the extent a provision of this Agreement is void or prohibited under applicable law, that provision shall be null and void and severed from the other terms of this Agreement. The remaining provisions shall be enforced to the fullest extent possible.
  B. The Dentist's waiver of one default does not waive any other default, whether the same or different, in the future.
  C. This Agreement is intended as the entire Agreement and replaces all prior and contemporaneous, written or oral, Agreements on the subject matter covered herein. The Agreement may only be modified by a written document signed by all parties to this Agreement.
  D. The terms "I," "me" and "my" includes each person who signs this Agreement, except the Dentist. If more than one person has signed this Agreement, each will be responsible for repaying the Obligations in full.

  I have received a copy of this Agreement.

NOTICE TO CUSTOMER	(a)	DO NOT SIGN THIS BEFORE YOU READ THE WRITING ON THE REVERSE SIDE, EVEN IF OTHERWISE ADVISED.
	(b)	DO NOT SIGN THIS IF IT CONTAINS ANY BLANK SPACES.
	(c)	YOU ARE ENTITLED TO AN EXACT COPY OF ANY AGREEMENT YOU SIGN.
	(d)	YOU HAVE THE RIGHT AT ANY TIME TO PAY IN ADVANCE THE UNPAID BALANCE DUE UNDER THIS AGREEMENT AND YOU MAY BE ENTITLED TO A PARTIAL REFUND OF FINANCE CHARGE.

Dated _____   X _____
                                                            Patient or patient's parent or legal guardian

_____   •
                Dentist   X _____ /
By _____   Print name
            Authorized Signature
Address: _____   •
                                                      X _____
_____   Print name

                                          Address: _____

                                          _____

                                          County: _____

Form No. T280FA   **FINANCIAL ARRANGEMENTS - U.S.**

117

Angelica Green

welcome

| | | | | | | |
PATIENT NUMBER

© 2003 Wisconsin Dental Association
(800) 243-4675

Date _____

Patient's Name _____   Date of Birth _____ ❏ Male ❏ Female
            Last   First   Initial

If Child: Parent's Name _____

How do you wish to be addressed _____
Single ❏ Married ❏ Separated ❏ Divorced ❏ Widowed ❏ Minor ❏

Residence - Street _____

City _____ State _____ Zip _____

Business Address _____

Telephone: Res. _____ Bus. _____

Fax _____ Cell Phone # _____

eMail _____

Patient/Parent Employed By _____

Present Position _____

How Long Held _____

Spouse/Parent Name _____

Spouse Employed By _____

Present Position _____

How Long Held _____

Who is Responsible for this account _____

Drivers License No. _____

Method of Payment: Insurance ❏ Cash ❏ Credit Card ❏

Purpose of Call _____

Other Family Members in this Practice _____

_____

Whom may we thank for this referral _____

Patient/parent Social Security No. _____

Spouse/Parent Social Security No. _____

Someone to notify in case of emergency not living with you _____

_____

DENTAL INSURANCE 1ST COVERAGE

Employee Name _____ Date of Birth _____
Employer Name _____ Yrs. _____
Name of Insurance Co. _____
Address _____
_____
Telephone _____
Program or policy # _____
Social Security No. _____
Union Local or Group _____

DENTAL INSURANCE 2ND COVERAGE

Employee Name _____ Date of Birth _____
Employer Name _____ Yrs. _____
Name of Insurance Co. _____
Address _____
_____
Telephone _____
Program or policy # _____
Social Security No. _____
Union Local or Group _____

CONSENT:
I consent to the diagnostic procedures and treatment by the dentist necessary for proper dental care.

I consent to the dentist's use and disclosure of my records (or my child's records) to carry out treatment, to obtain payment, and for those activities and health care operations that are related to treatment or payment.

I consent to the disclosure of my records (or my child's records) to the following persons who are involved in my care (or my child's care) or payment for that care.

_____

_____

My consent to disclosure of records shall be effective until I revoke it in writing.

I authorize payment directly to the dentist or dental group of insurance benefits otherwise payable to me. I understand that my dental care insurance carrier or payor of my dental benefits may pay less than the actual bill for services, and that I am financially responsible for payment in full of all accounts. By signing this statement, I revoke all previous agreements to the contrary and agree to be responsible for payment of services not paid, by my dental care payor.

I attest to the accuracy of the information on this page.

PATIENT'S OR GUARDIAN'S SIGNATURE

_____

DATE _____

Form No. T110R

REGISTRATION

Angelica Green

welcome

PATIENT NUMBER

Patient's Name _____
Last   First   Initial   Date of Birth

1. Purpose of initial visit _____
   _____
2. Are you aware of a problem?_____
   _____
3. How long since your last dental visit? _____
4. What was done at that time?_____
   _____
5. Previous dentist's name_____
   Address:_____ Tel. _____
6. When was the last time your teeth were cleaned?_____

CIRCLE THE APPROPRIATE ANSWER. IF YOU DON'T KNOW THE CORRECT ANSWER,
PLEASE WRITE "DON'T KNOW" ON THE LINE AFTER THE QUESTION.

7. Have you made regular visits? ....YES NO
   How often: _____
8. Were dental x-rays taken? ....YES NO
9. Have you lost any teeth or have any teeth been removed? ....YES NO
   Why?_____
10. Have they been replaced? ....YES NO
11. How have they been replaced?
    a. Fixed bridge _____ Age _____
    b. Removable bridge _____ Age _____
    c. Denture _____ Age _____
    d. Implant _____ Age _____
12. Are you unhappy with the replacement? ....YES NO
    If yes, explain _____
13. Would you like to know about permanent replacements? ....YES NO
14. Have you ever had any problems or complications with previous dental treatment? ...YES NO
    If yes, explain: _____
15. Do you clench or grind your teeth? ....YES NO
16. Does your jaw click or pop? ....YES NO
17. Have you experienced any pain or soreness in the muscles of your
    face or around your ear? ....YES NO
18. Do you have frequent headaches, neckaches or shoulder aches? ..YES NO
19. Does food get caught in your teeth? ....YES NO
20. Are any of your teeth sensitive to: ☐ Hot? ☐ Cold? ☐ Sweets? ☐ Pressure?
21. Do your gums bleed or hurt? ....YES NO
    When? _____
22. How often do you brush your teeth _____ When?_____
23. Do you use dental floss? ....YES NO
    How often?_____
24. Are any of your teeth loose, tipped, shifted or chipped? ....YES NO
25. Are you unhappy with the appearance of your teeth? ....YES NO
26. How do you feel about your teeth in general?_____
27. Do you feel your breath is offensive at times? ....YES NO
28. Have you ever had gum treatment or surgery? ....YES NO
    What?_____
    Where?_____
    When?_____
29. Have you had any orthodontic work?_____
30. Have you had any unpleasant dental experiences or is there anything about dentistry that you
    strongly dislike? _____
31. Do you have any questions or concerns? ....YES NO

I CERTIFY THAT THE ABOVE INFORMATION IS COMPLETE AND ACCURATE

PATIENT'S / GUARDIAN'S SIGNATURE _____ DATE_____

DENTIST'S SIGNATURE _____ DATE_____

COMMENTS

ANEST.

MED. ALERT

DENTAL HISTORY

Form No. T150DH

119

Angelica Green

PATIENT NUMBER

© 2004 Wisconsin Dental Association
(800) 243-4675

welcome

Patient's Name _____

Last   First   Initial   Date of Birth

CIRCLE THE APPROPRIATE ANSWER, IF YOU DON'T KNOW THE CORRECT ANSWER PLEASE WRITE "DON'T KNOW" ON THE LINE AFTER THE QUESTION

COMMENTS

1. Physician's Name_____
   Address_____
   _____ Tel:(___)_____
2. Are you under a physician's care? . . . . YES NO
   Since when_____Why_____
3. When was your last complete physical exam?_____
4. Are you taking any medication or substances? . . . . YES NO
   (If yes, please list medications in comments section or on the back of this form.)
5. Do you routinely take health related substances? (Vitamins, herbal supplements, natural products) . . YES NO
6. Are you allergic to any medications or substances? (please list) . . . . YES NO
7. Do you have any other allergies or hives? . . . . YES NO
8. Do you have any problems with penicillin, antibiotics, anesthetics
   or other medications? . . . . YES NO
9. Are you sensitive to any metals or latex? . . . . YES NO
10. Are you pregnant or suspect you may be? . . . . YES NO
11. Do you use any birth control medications? . . . . YES NO
12. Have you ever been treated for or been told you might have heart disease? . . . . YES NO
13. Do you have a pacemaker, an artificial heart valve implant, or
    been diagnosed with mitral valve prolapse? . . . . YES NO
14. Have you ever had rheumatic fever? . . . . YES NO
15. Are you aware of any heart murmurs? . . . . YES NO
16. Do you have high or low blood pressure? (please circle) . . . . YES NO
17. Have you ever had a serious illness or major surgery? . . . . YES NO
    If so, explain_____
18. Have you ever had radiation treatment, chemo treatment for tumor
    growth or other condition? . . . . YES NO
19. Do you have inflammatory diseases, such as arthritis or rheumatism? . . . . YES NO
20. Do you have any artificial joints/prosthesis? . . . . YES NO
21. Do you have any blood disorders, such as anemia, leukemia, etc? . . . . YES NO
22. Have you ever bled excessively after being cut or injured? . . . . YES NO
23. Do you have any stomach problems? . . . . YES NO
24. Do you have any kidney problems? . . . . YES NO
25. Do you have any liver problems? . . . . YES NO
26. Are you diabetic? . . . . YES NO
27. Do you have fainting or dizzy spells? . . . . YES NO
28. Do you have asthma? . . . . YES NO
29. Do you have epilepsy or seizure disorder? . . . . YES NO
30. Do you or have you had venereal disease? . . . . YES NO
31. Have you tested HIV positive? . . . . YES NO
32. Do you have AIDS? . . . . YES NO
33. Have you had or do you test positive for hepatitis? . . . . YES NO
34. Do you or have you had T.B.? . . . . YES NO
35. Do you smoke, chew, use snuff or any other forms of tobacco? . . . . YES NO
36. Do you regularly consume more than one or two alcoholic beverages a day? . . . . . YES NO
37. Do you habitually use controlled substances? . . . . YES NO
38. Have you had psychiatric treatment? . . . . YES NO
39. Have you taken any prescription drugs fenfluramine, fenfluramine combined with
    phentermine (fen-phen), dexfenfluramine (redux), or other weight loss products? . . . . . YES NO
40. Do you have any disease condition, or problem not listed? If so, explain_____

41. Is there anything else we should know about your health that we have not covered in this form?

42. Would you like to speak to the Doctor privately about any problem? . . . . YES NO

I CERTIFY THAT THE ABOVE INFORMATION IS COMPLETE AND ACCURATE

PATIENT'S / GUARDIAN'S SIGNATURE_____ DATE_____

DENTIST'S SIGNATURE_____ DATE_____

ANEST.

MED. ALERT

MEDICAL HISTORY

Form No. T140MH

120

Angelica Green

× ☐☐☐☐☐☐ ×
PATIENT NUMBER

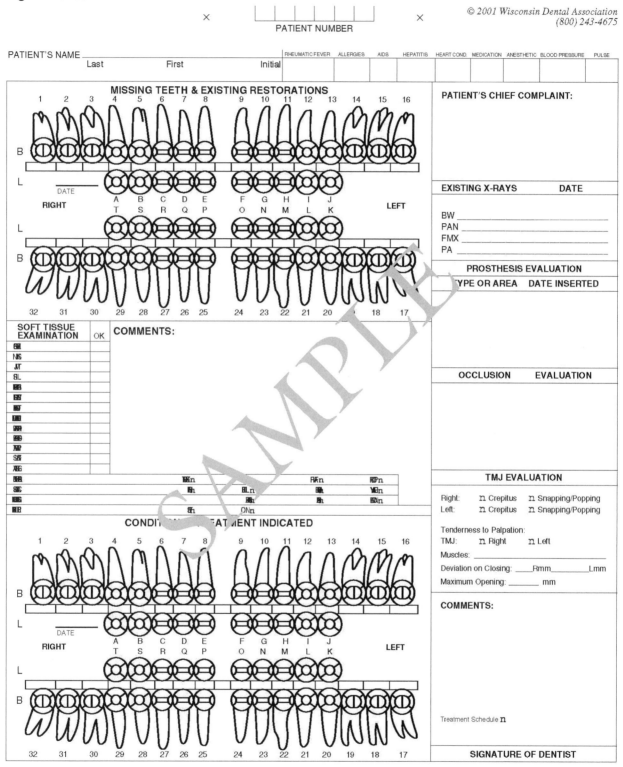

PATIENT'S NAME _____
Last   First   Initial

RHEUMATIC FEVER	ALLERGIES	AIDS	HEPATITIS	HEART COND.	MEDICATION	ANESTHETIC	BLOOD PRESSURE	PULSE

MISSING TEETH & EXISTING RESTORATIONS

PATIENT'S CHIEF COMPLAINT:

EXISTING X-RAYS   DATE

BW _____
PAN _____
FMX _____
PA _____

PROSTHESIS EVALUATION
TYPE OR AREA   DATE INSERTED

SOFT TISSUE EXAMINATION | OK | COMMENTS:

OCCLUSION   EVALUATION

CONDITIONS & TREATMENT INDICATED

TMJ EVALUATION

Right: n Crepitus   n Snapping/Popping
Left: n Crepitus   n Snapping/Popping

Tenderness to Palpation:
TMJ: n Right   n Left
Muscles: _____
Deviation on Closing: ____Rmm_____Lmm
Maximum Opening: _____ mm

COMMENTS:

Treatment Schedule n

SIGNATURE OF DENTIST

Form No. T170CE

CLINICAL EXAMINATION

Angelica Green

× ⊞⊞⊞⊞⊞⊞ ×   ⊞⊞

© 2001 Wisconsin Dental Association
(800) 243-4675

PATIENT'S NAME _____

| Last | First | Initial | Date of Birth |

DATE _____ THERAPIST _____

PROBING – Place probe as close to the contact point as possible, directed along the long axis of the tooth. Take the mesial, mid and distal measurements from the buccal aspect. Repeat for lingual aspect. Record only those measurements over 3mm.
BLEEDING – After probing each quadrant, note whether or not bleeding has occurred. Indicate the bleeding area by circling the pocket in red.
MOBILITY – Move each tooth between two instrument handles in a bucco-lingual direction and attempt to depress each tooth in its socket. Grade each tooth accordingly: 0 - Movement of less than 0.5mm; 1 - 0.5mm to 1.0mm; 2 - 1.0mm to 2.0mm; 3 - Movement of more that 2.0mm or depressible.
FURCATION – Probe from the buccal and lingual. Record accordingly: 0 - Normal; 1 - Slight; 2 - Moderate; 3 - Through and through.
RECESSION – Measure the exposed surface from the cemental enamel junction (CEJ) to the gingival crest. Enter the distance in millimeters (mm).

R

SAMPLE

L

(Periodontal charting grid for teeth 1–16 and 32–17, with rows for Pocket Depth B/L, Mobility, Furcation, Recession)

| Enter highest POCKET DEPTH score in appropriate box | ☐ Any pocket depth reading from 3 to 5mm, read below | ☐ Any pocket depth reading over 5mm, read below |
| Enter highest MOBILITY SCORE in appropriate box | ☐ Any mobility of 1, read below | ☐ Any mobility of 2 or 3, read below |

BLEEDING — ☐ When any bleeding upon probing is noted, read below

INSTRUMENTS FOR TREATMENT SELECTION — Locate square containing score farthest to the right and follow treatment, listed below.

Gingivitis
☐ Explanation of periodontal disease.
A. Hygienist Treatment
1. Oral Hygiene Instruction
2. Prophylaxis

Moderate Periodontitis
OPTION 1
A. Dentist or Hygienist Treatment
1. Oral Hygiene Instruction
2. Periodontal Root Planing
3. Occlusal Analysis
4. Maintenance Recall
OPTION 2
B. Referral to Periodontist

Advanced Periodontitis
OPTION 1
A. Referral to Periodontist
OPTION 2
B. Dentist Treatment
1. Oral Hygiene Instruction
2. Periodontal Root Planing
3. Occlusal Analysis
4. Periodontal Surgery
5. Splinting
6. Maintenance Recall

Form No. T181PS **PERIODONTAL SCREENING EXAMINATION**

122

Appendix

Copyright © 2007, 2000 by Saunders, an imprint of Elsevier, Inc. All rights reserved.

Angelica Green

| | | | | | | |

PATIENT NUMBER

PATIENT'S NAME _____

| Last | First | Initial | Date |

DATE	TREATMENT PLAN	FEE	ALTERNATE TREATMENT	FEE	PROB # ASGN

RELEASE:

I accept the above treatment plan. I understand that because of unexpected circumstances, the treatment, the fees for treatment and/or the materials required as explained to me at this time, may require some changes after actual care has begun.

PATIENT'S/GUARDIAN'S SIGNATURE _____ DATE _____

ANEST.		MED. ALERT

Form No. T201TP

TREATMENT PLAN

Angelica Green ✕ 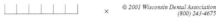 ✕   *© 2001 Wisconsin Dental Association*
(800) 243-4675

PATIENT'S NAME_____

　　　　　　　　　　　　　Last　　　　　　　　　First　　　　　　　　Initial

AGREEMENT TO PAY FOR DENTAL SERVICES

Agreement to Pay. For services rendered or to be rendered to me, or to others at my request, I promise to pay to Dentist $_____, plus interest and other charges as stated below ("Obligations"). I will make the payments described in the payment schedule to Dentist at the address shown on the opposite side of this form.

Federally Required Disclosures. The calculations shown below are computed on the assumption that each payment will be made in full on the date due:

ITEMIZATION OF AMOUNT FINANCED

　　Dental Fees　　　　Down Payment　　　Amount Financed

　　$ _____ – $ _____ = $ _____

ANNUAL PERCENTAGE RATE The cost of your credit as a yearly rate. _____%	FINANCE CHARGE The dollar amount the credit will cost you. $_____	Amount Financed The amount of credit provided to you or on your behalf. $_____	Total of Payments The amount you will have paid after you have made all payments as scheduled. $_____	Total Sale Price The total cost of your purchase on credit, including your downpayment of $_____ $_____

Your payment schedule will be: _____ equal consecutive installments of $ _____ each, and one final installment of _____ on the _____ day of each successive month beginning_____ , 19_____.

　Late Charge. If a payment is not paid on or before the 10th day after the due date, I may be charge[...]0[...] or 5.00% of th[...] unpaid amount, whichever is less.
　If I pay off early, I will not have to pay a penalty, and I may be entitled to a refund of unearned finance cha[...]
　See your contract documents for any additional information about nonpayments [...] default, any required repay[...] before the scheduled date, and prepayment refunds and penalties.

Other Charges. I agree to pay a charge of _____ for each check [...] sented for pay[...]ent and returned unpaid. I also agree to pay all costs of collection, to the extent not proh[...]ed under

Application of Payments. Unless otherwise required [...] applicab[...] law, payme[...] [...]ll be applied as directed by Dentist.

Default and Remedies. I will be in default of [...]y Obligatio[...] under this Agreement if I have an amount outstanding which exceeds one full payment which has [...]ained unpaid [...] more than 10 days after the scheduled or deferred due dates; or the first or last payment is not p[...] [...]ithin 40 days o[...] [...] due date.

In the event of default, the Dentist shall:

　A. Have all the rights and remedies provided by la[...] [...]d this Agreement. All remedies shall be cumulative and __ the exercise of one shall [...] [...]revent the e[...]ercise o[...] [...] other remedies.

　B. Upon default the Dentist may[...] a[...] [...] [...]ption, accelerate the amount due, without notice. In that event, the Obligations shall become p[...]vable a[...] [...]tice is provided and the right to cure has expired.

Miscellaneous.

　A. To the exten[...] [...]vision of this [...] [...]ement is void or prohibited under applicable law, that provision shall be null and void an[...] [...]red from [...]e other terms of this Agreement. The remaining provisions shall be enforced to the [...]llest[...] exte[...] [...]ible.

　B. The Dentist's wa[...] of one [...]ault does not waive any other default, whether the same or different, in the [...]ture.

　C. This Agreement is [...]tended as the entire Agreement and replaces all prior and contemporaneous, written or oral, Agreements o[...] the subject matter covered herein. The Agreement may only be modified by a written [...] [...]d by [...] parties to this Agreement.

　D. [...] [...]rms "I[...] [...]e" and "my" includes each person who signs this Agreement, except the Dentist. If more than one pers[...] has signed this Agreement, each will be responsible for repaying the Obligations in full.

　I have received a copy of this Agreement.

NOTICE TO CUSTOMER	(a)	DO NOT SIGN THIS BEFORE YOU READ THE WRITING ON THE REVERSE SIDE, EVEN IF OTHERWISE ADVISED.
	(b)	DO NOT SIGN THIS IF IT CONTAINS ANY BLANK SPACES.
	(c)	YOU ARE ENTITLED TO AN EXACT COPY OF ANY AGREEMENT YOU SIGN.
	(d)	YOU HAVE THE RIGHT AT ANY TIME TO PAY IN ADVANCE THE UNPAID BALANCE DUE UNDER THIS AGREEMENT AND YOU MAY BE ENTITLED TO A PARTIAL REFUND OF FINANCE CHARGE.

Dated _____　　　　X _____
　　　　　　　　　　　　　　　　　　　　　　Patient or patient's parent or legal guardian
　　　　　　　　　　　　　　　　　　　　• _____
_____　　　　　　　　　　Print name
　　　　　　　Dentist

By _____　　X _____ /
　　　Authorized Signature
Address: _____　　• _____
　　　　　　　　　　　　　　　　　　　　　　　　　Print name
_____　　Address: _____

　　　　　　　　　　　　　　　　　　　_____

　　　　　　　　　　　　　　　　　　　County: _____

Form No. T280FA   **FINANCIAL ARRANGEMENTS - U.S.**

Holly Barry

© 2003 Wisconsin Dental Association
(800) 243-4675

welcome

PATIENT NUMBER

Date _____

Patient's Name _____   Date of Birth _____ ❑ Male ❑ Female
Last   First   Initial

If Child: Parent's Name _____

How do you wish to be addressed _____
Single ❑   Married ❑   Separated ❑   Divorced ❑   Widowed ❑   Minor ❑

Residence - Street _____

City _____ State _____ Zip _____

Business Address _____

Telephone: Res. _____ Bus. _____

Fax _____ Cell Phone # _____

eMail _____

Patient/Parent Employed By _____

Present Position _____

How Long Held _____

Spouse/Parent Name _____

Spouse Employed By _____

Present Position _____

How Long Held _____

Who is Responsible for this account _____

Drivers License No. _____

Method of Payment: Insurance ❑   Cash ❑   Credit Card ❑

Purpose of Call _____

Other Family Members in this Practice _____

Whom may we thank for this referral _____

Patient/parent Social Security No. _____

Spouse/Parent Social Security No. _____

Someone to notify in case of emergency not living with you _____

DENTAL INSURANCE 1ST COVERAGE

Employee Name _____ Date of Birth _____
Employer Name _____ Yrs. _____
Name of Insurance Co. _____
Address _____
_____
Telephone _____
Program or policy # _____
Social Security No. _____
Union Local or Group _____

DENTAL INSURANCE 2ND COVERAGE

Employee Name _____ Date of Birth _____
Employer Name _____ Yrs. _____
Name of Insurance Co. _____
Address _____
_____
Telephone _____
Program or policy # _____
Social Security No. _____
Union Local or Group _____

CONSENT:

I consent to the diagnostic procedures and treatment by the dentist necessary for proper dental care.

I consent to the dentist's use and disclosure of my records (or my child's records) to carry out treatment, to obtain payment, and for those activities and health care operations that are related to treatment or payment.

I consent to the disclosure of my records (or my child's records) to the following persons who are involved in my care (or my child's care) or payment for that care.

_____
_____

My consent to disclosure of records shall be effective until I revoke it in writing.

I authorize payment directly to the dentist or dental group of insurance benefits otherwise payable to me. I understand that my dental care insurance carrier or payor of my dental benefits may pay less than the actual bill for services, and that I am financially responsible for payment in full of all accounts. By signing this statement, I revoke all previous agreements to the contrary and agree to be responsible for payment of services not paid, by my dental care payor.

I attest to the accuracy of the information on this page.

PATIENT'S OR GUARDIAN'S SIGNATURE

_____

DATE _____

Form No. T110R

REGISTRATION

Holly Barry

× | | | | | | | | ×
PATIENT NUMBER

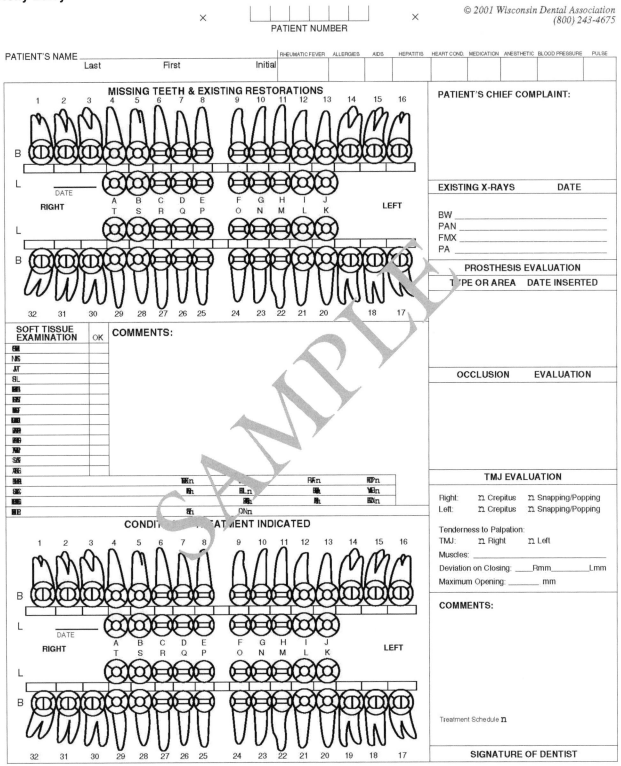

PATIENT'S NAME _____
Last   First   Initial

RHEUMATIC FEVER	ALLERGIES	AIDS	HEPATITIS	HEART COND.	MEDICATION	ANESTHETIC	BLOOD PRESSURE	PULSE

MISSING TEETH & EXISTING RESTORATIONS

PATIENT'S CHIEF COMPLAINT:

EXISTING X-RAYS   DATE

BW _____
PAN _____
FMX _____
PA _____

PROSTHESIS EVALUATION

TYPE OR AREA   DATE INSERTED

OCCLUSION   EVALUATION

SOFT TISSUE EXAMINATION	OK

COMMENTS:

TMJ EVALUATION

Right: ∏ Crepitus   ∏ Snapping/Popping
Left: ∏ Crepitus   ∏ Snapping/Popping

Tenderness to Palpation:
TMJ: ∏ Right   ∏ Left
Muscles: _____
Deviation on Closing: ____Rmm_____Lmm
Maximum Opening: _____ mm

COMMENTS:

CONDITIONS / TREATMENT INDICATED

RIGHT   LEFT

Treatment Schedule ∏

SIGNATURE OF DENTIST

CLINICAL EXAMINATION

Form No. T170CE

Holly Barry

PATIENT NUMBER

PATIENT'S NAME _____

| Last | First | Initial | Date |

DATE	TREATMENT PLAN	FEE	ALTERNATE TREATMENT	FEE	PROB # ASGN

RELEASE:

I accept the above treatment plan. I understand that because of unexpected circumstances, the treatment, the fees for treatment and/or the materials required as explained to me at this time, may require some changes after actual care has begun.

PATIENT'S/GUARDIAN'S SIGNATURE _____ DATE _____

ANEST.

MED. ALERT

Form No. T201TP

TREATMENT PLAN

127

Appendix

Holly Barry × | | | | | | × © 2001 Wisconsin Dental Association
(800) 243-4675

PATIENT'S NAME_____

Last   First   Initial

AGREEMENT TO PAY FOR DENTAL SERVICES

Agreement to Pay. For services rendered or to be rendered to me, or to others at my request, I promise to pay to Dentist $_____, plus interest and other charges as stated below ("Obligations"). I will make the payments described in the payment schedule to Dentist at the address shown on the opposite side of this form.

Federally Required Disclosures. The calculations shown below are computed on the assumption that each payment will be made in full on the date due.

ITEMIZATION OF AMOUNT FINANCED

Dental Fees	Down Payment	Amount Financed
$ _____	– $ _____	= $ _____

ANNUAL PERCENTAGE RATE	FINANCE CHARGE	Amount Financed	Total of Payments	Total Sale Price
The cost of your credit as a yearly rate.	The dollar amount the credit will cost you.	The amount of credit provided to you or on your behalf.	The amount you will have paid after you have made all payments as scheduled.	The total cost of your purchase on credit, including your downpayment of $_____
_____ %	$_____	$_____	$_____	$_____

Your payment schedule will be: _____ equal consecutive installments of $ _____ each, and one final installment of _____ on the _____ day of each successive month beginning_____, 19_____.

Late Charge. If a payment is not paid on or before the 10th day after the due date, I may be charged ____ or 5.00% of the unpaid amount, whichever is less.

If I pay off early, I will not have to pay a penalty, and I may be entitled to a refund of unearned finance charges.

See your contract documents for any additional information about nonpayment, default, any required repayment in full before the scheduled date, and prepayment refunds and penalties.

Other Charges. I agree to pay a charge of _____ for each check presented for payment and returned unpaid. I also agree to pay all costs of collection, to the extent not prohibited under ____.

Application of Payments. Unless otherwise required by applicable law, payment will be applied as directed by Dentist.

Default and Remedies. I will be in default of my Obligation under this Agreement if I have an amount outstanding which exceeds one full payment which has remained unpaid for more than 10 days after the scheduled or deferred due dates; or the first or last payment is not paid within 40 days of due date.

In the event of default, the Dentist shall:
A. Have all the rights and remedies provided by law and this Agreement. All remedies shall be cumulative and __ the exercise of one shall prevent the exercise of other remedies.

B. Upon default the Dentist may, at its option, accelerate the amount due, without notice. In that event, the Obligations shall become payable after notice is provided and the right to cure has expired.

Miscellaneous.
A. To the extent any provision of this Agreement is void or prohibited under applicable law, that provision shall be null and void and severed from the other terms of this Agreement. The remaining provisions shall be enforced to the fullest extent possible.
B. The Dentist's waiver of one default does not waive any other default, whether the same or different, in the future.
C. This Agreement is intended as the entire Agreement and replaces all prior and contemporaneous, written or oral, Agreements on the subject matter covered herein. The Agreement may only be modified by a written signed by parties to this Agreement.
D. The terms "I", "me" and "my" includes each person who signs this Agreement, except the Dentist. If more than one person has signed this Agreement, each will be responsible for repaying the Obligations in full.

I have received a copy of this Agreement.

NOTICE TO CUSTOMER	(a)	DO NOT SIGN THIS BEFORE YOU READ THE WRITING ON THE REVERSE SIDE, EVEN IF OTHERWISE ADVISED.
	(b)	DO NOT SIGN THIS IF IT CONTAINS ANY BLANK SPACES.
	(c)	YOU ARE ENTITLED TO AN EXACT COPY OF ANY AGREEMENT YOU SIGN.
	(d)	YOU HAVE THE RIGHT AT ANY TIME TO PAY IN ADVANCE THE UNPAID BALANCE DUE UNDER THIS AGREEMENT AND YOU MAY BE ENTITLED TO A PARTIAL REFUND OF FINANCE CHARGE.

Dated _____

X _____
Patient or patient's parent or legal guardian

_____
Dentist

_____
Print name

By _____
Authorized Signature

X _____ /

Address: _____

_____
Print name

Address: _____

_____

County: _____

Form No. T280FA

FINANCIAL ARRANGEMENTS - U.S.

128

Appendix

Lynn Bacca

PATIENT NUMBER

welcome

Date _____

Patient's Name_____

Last   First   Initial

Date of Birth _____ ❏ Male ❏ Female

If Child: Parent's Name_____

How do you wish to be addressed _____
Single ❏   Married ❏   Separated ❏   Divorced ❏   Widowed ❏   Minor ❏

Residence - Street _____

City_____ State _____ Zip _____

Business Address _____

Telephone: Res. _____ Bus. _____

Fax _____ Cell Phone #_____

eMail _____

Patient/Parent Employed By _____

Present Position _____

How Long Held _____

Spouse/Parent Name _____

Spouse Employed By _____

Present Position _____

How Long Held _____

Who is Responsible for this account _____

Drivers License No. _____

Method of Payment: Insurance ❏   Cash ❏   Credit Card ❏

Purpose of Call _____

Other Family Members in this Practice _____

_____

Whom may we thank for this referral _____

Patient/parent Social Security No. _____

Spouse/Parent Social Security No. _____

Someone to notify in case of emergency not living with you _____

_____

DENTAL INSURANCE 1ST COVERAGE

Employee Name _____ Date of Birth _____
Employer Name _____ Yrs. _____
Name of Insurance Co. _____
Address _____
_____
Telephone _____
Program or policy # _____
Social Security No. _____
Union Local or Group _____

DENTAL INSURANCE 2ND COVERAGE

Employee Name _____ Date of Birth _____
Employer Name _____ Yrs. _____
Name of Insurance Co. _____
Address _____
_____
Telephone _____
Program or policy # _____
Social Security No. _____
Union Local or Group _____

CONSENT:
I consent to the diagnostic procedures and treatment by the dentist necessary for proper dental care.

I consent to the dentist's use and disclosure of my records (or my child's records) to carry out treatment, to obtain payment, and for those activities and health care operations that are related to treatment or payment.

I consent to the disclosure of my records (or my child's records) to the following persons who are involved in my care (or my child's care) or payment for that care.

_____

My consent to disclosure of records shall be effective until I revoke it in writing.

I authorize payment directly to the dentist or dental group of insurance benefits otherwise payable to me. I understand that my dental care insurance carrier or payor of my dental benefits may pay less than the actual bill for services, and that I am financially responsible for payment in full of all accounts. By signing this statement, I revoke all previous agreements to the contrary and agree to be responsible for payment of services not paid, by my dental care payor.

I attest to the accuracy of the information on this page.

PATIENT'S OR GUARDIAN'S SIGNATURE

_____

DATE _____

SAMPLE

Form No. T110R

REGISTRATION

Lynn Bacca

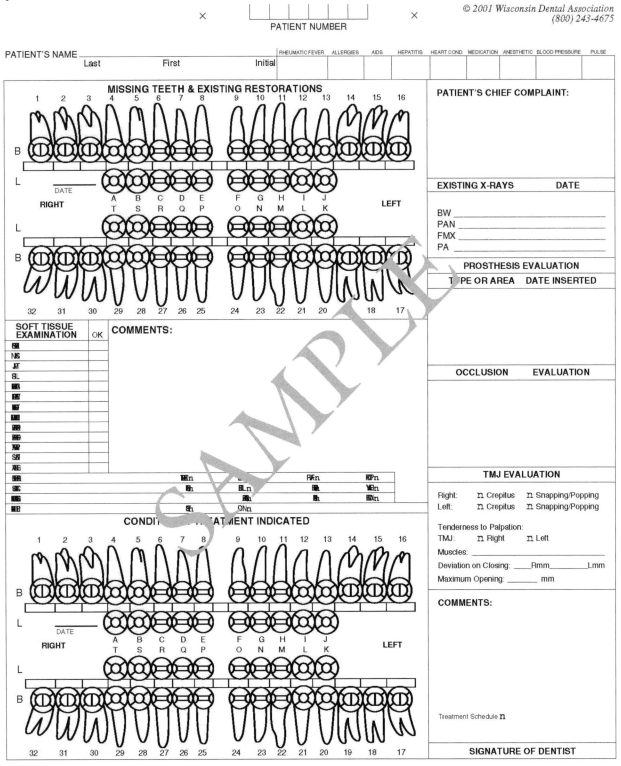

× | | | | | | | | ×

PATIENT NUMBER

PATIENT'S NAME _____

Last   First   Initial

RHEUMATIC FEVER	ALLERGIES	AIDS	HEPATITIS	HEART COND.	MEDICATION	ANESTHETIC	BLOOD PRESSURE	PULSE

MISSING TEETH & EXISTING RESTORATIONS

PATIENT'S CHIEF COMPLAINT:

EXISTING X-RAYS   DATE

BW _____
PAN _____
FMX _____
PA _____

PROSTHESIS EVALUATION
TYPE OR AREA   DATE INSERTED

SOFT TISSUE EXAMINATION

COMMENTS:

OCCLUSION   EVALUATION

TMJ EVALUATION

Right: ∏ Crepitus   ∏ Snapping/Popping
Left: ∏ Crepitus   ∏ Snapping/Popping

Tenderness to Palpation:
TMJ: ∏ Right   ∏ Left
Muscles: _____
Deviation on Closing: ____Rmm_____Lmm
Maximum Opening: _____ mm

COMMENTS:

CONDITION & TREATMENT INDICATED

Treatment Schedule ∏

SIGNATURE OF DENTIST

Form No. T170CE

CLINICAL EXAMINATION

Lynn Bacca

PATIENT NUMBER

PATIENT'S NAME _____

| | Last | First | Initial | Date |

DATE	TREATMENT PLAN	FEE	ALTERNATE TREATMENT	FEE	PROB # ASGN

RELEASE:

I accept the above treatment plan. I understand that because of unexpected circumstances, the treatment, the fees for treatment and/or the materials required as explained to me at this time, may require some changes after actual care has begun.

PATIENT'S/GUARDIAN'S SIGNATURE _____ DATE _____

| ANEST. | | MED. ALERT |

Form No. T201TP

TREATMENT PLAN

131

Lynn Bacca   × | | | | | | | ×   *© 2001 Wisconsin Dental Association*
(800) 243-4675

PATIENT'S NAME_____
Last   First   Initial

AGREEMENT TO PAY FOR DENTAL SERVICES

Agreement to Pay. For services rendered or to be rendered to me, or to others at my request, I promise to pay to Dentist $_____, plus interest and other charges as stated below ("Obligations"). I will make the payments described in the payment schedule to Dentist at the address shown on the opposite side of this form.

Federally Required Disclosures. The calculations shown below are computed on the assumption that each payment will be made in full on the date due:

ITEMIZATION OF AMOUNT FINANCED

Dental Fees   Down Payment   Amount Financed

$ _____ – $ _____ = $ _____

ANNUAL PERCENTAGE RATE	FINANCE CHARGE	Amount Financed	Total of Payments	Total Sale Price
The cost of your credit as a yearly rate.	The dollar amount the credit will cost you.	The amount of credit provided to you or on your behalf.	The amount you will have paid after you have made all payments as scheduled.	The total cost of your purchase on credit, including your downpayment of $_____
_____%	$_____	$_____	$_____	$_____

Your payment schedule will be: _____ equal consecutive installments of $ _____ each, and one final installment of _____ on the _____ day of each successive month beginning_____, 19_____.

Late Charge. If a payment is not paid on or before the 10th day after the due date, I may be charged $10.00 or 5.00% of the unpaid amount, whichever is less.
If I pay off early, I will not have to pay a penalty, and I may be entitled to a refund of unearned finance charges.
See your contract documents for any additional information about nonpayments, default, any required repayment in full before the scheduled date, and prepayment refunds and penalties.

Other Charges. I agree to pay a charge of _____ for each check presented for payment and returned unpaid. I also agree to pay all costs of collection, to the extent not prohibited under law.

Application of Payments. Unless otherwise required by applicable law, payments will be applied as directed by Dentist.

Default and Remedies. I will be in default of my Obligations under this Agreement if I have an amount outstanding which exceeds one full payment which has remained unpaid for more than 10 days after the scheduled or deferred due dates; or the first or last payment is not paid within 40 days its due date.

In the event of default, the Dentist shall:
A. Have all the rights and remedies provided by law and this Agreement. All remedies shall be cumulative and ___ the exercise of one shall not prevent the exercise of other remedies.

B. Upon default the Dentist may, at its option, accelerate the amount due, without notice. In that event, the Obligations shall become payable and notice is provided and the right to cure has expired.

Miscellaneous.
A. To the extent a provision of this Agreement is void or prohibited under applicable law, that provision shall be null and void and severed from the other terms of this Agreement. The remaining provisions shall be enforced to the fullest extent possible.
B. The Dentist's waiver of one default does not waive any other default, whether the same or different, in the future.
C. This Agreement is intended as the entire Agreement and replaces all prior and contemporaneous, written or oral, Agreements on the subject matter covered herein. The Agreement may only be modified by a written agreement signed by parties to this Agreement.
D. The terms "I", "me" and "my" includes each person who signs this Agreement, except the Dentist. If more than one person has signed this Agreement, each will be responsible for repaying the Obligations in full.

I have received a copy of this Agreement.

NOTICE TO CUSTOMER	(a)	DO NOT SIGN THIS BEFORE YOU READ THE WRITING ON THE REVERSE SIDE, EVEN IF OTHERWISE ADVISED.
	(b)	DO NOT SIGN THIS IF IT CONTAINS ANY BLANK SPACES.
	(c)	YOU ARE ENTITLED TO AN EXACT COPY OF ANY AGREEMENT YOU SIGN.
	(d)	YOU HAVE THE RIGHT AT ANY TIME TO PAY IN ADVANCE THE UNPAID BALANCE DUE UNDER THIS AGREEMENT AND YOU MAY BE ENTITLED TO A PARTIAL REFUND OF FINANCE CHARGE.

Dated _____   X_____
                                       Patient or patient's parent or legal guardian
                                       •
_____   _____
Dentist   Print name
By _____   X_____ /
   Authorized Signature
Address: _____   •_____
                                       Print name
_____   Address: _____

                                       _____

                                       County: _____

Form No. T280FA   # FINANCIAL ARRANGEMENTS - U.S.

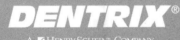
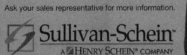
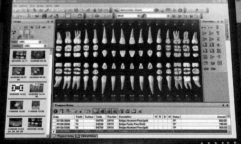